GETTING STARTED WITH THE PRIMARY SCLEROSING CHOLANGITIS DIET

Discover PSC-Friendly Recipes to Manage Symptoms, Prevent Liver Damage, and Eliminate Complications

Chris Preston, RDN

ACKNOWLEDGEMENTS

I would like to express my deepest gratitude to everyone who supported me throughout the journey of creating this book. To my family and friends, your unwavering encouragement and patience have been invaluable.

A special thanks to my team, whose expertise and guidance were crucial in developing the dietary plans and recipes shared in this book. Your insights have been a cornerstone of this work.

I am also deeply grateful to my editor, Michael Jones, for your meticulous attention to detail and for helping shape this book into a comprehensive and accessible guide.

To the support groups and communities who shared their experiences and provided feedback, your contributions have enriched this book and made it more relatable for those living with fructose intolerance.

Lastly, to my readers, thank you for embarking on this journey with me. I hope this book provides you with the knowledge and tools to navigate your dietary needs and improve your quality of life.

COPYRIGHT

Copyright © Chris Preston, RDN. All rights reserved.

No part of this publication may be reproduced, distributed, or transmitted in any form or by any means, including photocopying, recording, or other electronic or mechanical methods, without the prior written permission of the publisher, except in the case of brief quotations embodied in critical reviews and certain other noncommercial uses permitted by copyright law.

This book is intended to provide general information about diet and nutrition. It is not intended as a substitute for professional medical advice, diagnosis, or treatment. Always seek the advice of your physician or other qualified health provider with any questions you may have regarding a medical condition.

TABLE OF CONTENTS

PART I

UNDERSTANDING PRIMARY SCLEROSING CHOLANGITIS (PSC)

Primary sclerosing cholangitis (PSC) (skluh-ROHS-ing) cholangitis (koh-lan-JIE-tis) is a chronic, or long-term, disease that slowly damages the bile ducts. Bile is a digestive liquid that is made in the liver. It travels through the bile ducts to the gallbladder and the small intestine, where it helps digest fats and fatty vitamins.

In patients with PSC, the bile ducts become blocked due to inflammation and scarring or fibrosis. This causes bile to accumulate in the liver, where it gradually damages liver cells and causes cirrhosis, or fibrosis of the liver. As cirrhosis progresses and the amount of scar tissue in the liver increases, the liver slowly loses its ability to function. The scar tissue may block drainage of the bile ducts leading to infection of the bile. . A majority of people with primary sclerosing cholangitis also have inflammatory bowel disease, such as ulcerative colitis or Crohn's disease.

PSC advances very slowly. Many patients may have the disease for years before symptoms develop. Symptoms may remain at a stable level, they may come and go, or they may progress gradually. Liver failure may occur 10-15 years after diagnosis, but this may take even longer for some PSC patients. Many people with PSC will ultimately need a liver transplant, typically about 10 years after being diagnosed with the disease. PSC may also lead to bile duct cancer. Endoscopy and MRI tests may be done to monitor the disease. Care for primary sclerosing cholangitis focuses on monitoring liver function, managing symptoms and, when possible, doing procedures that temporarily open blocked bile ducts.

Is primary sclerosing cholangitis serious?

Yes. While you might not have symptoms at first, PSC is a progressive disease that gets worse over time. When bile stalls in your bile ducts (cholestasis), it can begin to leak bile toxins into your bloodstream, which makes you sick. It also does progressive damage to your liver. Within 10 to 15 years, this can lead to liver failure. You can't live without a liver. While there are temporizing treatments, there is currently no cure for PSC, except a liver transplant.

What is the difference between primary sclerosing cholangitis and secondary sclerosing cholangitis?

"Primary" means that this disease is the original cause of inflammation and scarring of your bile ducts. There's no other cause but the disease. In secondary sclerosing cholangitis, inflammation (cholangitis) and scarring (sclerosis) of your bile ducts are secondary effects caused by something else. Some causes of secondary sclerosing cholangitis include:

Bile duct injury (for example, during surgery).

Infections of the bile ducts.

Chemotherapy.

Gallstones in your bile ducts.

Recurring pancreatitis.

What is the difference between primary biliary cirrhosis and primary sclerosing cholangitis?

Primary biliary cholangitis (PBC) is the current name for what was previously called primary biliary cirrhosis.

PBC and PSC are both progressive bile duct-related liver diseases, with similar symptoms and effects. Both diseases cause the gradual deterioration of your bile ducts. Destruction and scarring in your bile ducts cause them to narrow and the flow of bile to stall. The bile begins to back up into your liver, where it causes further damage. This leads to scarring and eventually, cirrhosis of the liver.

Here are the primary differences:

PBC only affects the bile ducts within your liver (intrahepatic), while PSC can affect the bile ducts inside or outside of your liver (extrahepatic).

PBC is more predominant in people assigned female at birth, by a ratio of 10:1. PSC is more predominant in people assigned male at birth, by a ratio of 2:1.

PSC is highly associated with preexisting IBD (80%), while PBC is not.

PSC is associated with an increased risk of developing bile duct cancer, while PBC is not.

PBC treatment involves using ursodeoxycholic acid (UDCA) to slow its progression. PSC currently has no medical treatment.

How common is this condition?

PSC is rare. It's estimated to occur in about 1 in 10,000 people worldwide.

Who does it affect?

PSC occurs in people assigned male at birth twice as often as in people assigned female at birth. It's most often diagnosed around the age of 40. About 80% of people with PSC also have inflammatory bowel disease, most often ulcerative colitis. It's more likely to occur in people with a family history of the disease.

Causes and Risk Factors

Causes

It's not clear what causes primary sclerosing cholangitis. An immune system reaction to an infection or toxin may trigger the disease in people who are genetically predisposed to it.

A large proportion of people with primary sclerosing cholangitis also have inflammatory bowel disease, an umbrella term that includes ulcerative colitis and Crohn's disease.

Primary sclerosing cholangitis and inflammatory bowel disease don't always appear at the same time, though. In some cases, primary sclerosing cholangitis is present for years before inflammatory bowel disease occurs. If primary sclerosing cholangitis is diagnosed, it's important to look for inflammatory bowel disease because there is a greater risk of colon cancer.

Somewhat less often, people being treated for inflammatory bowel disease turn out to have primary sclerosing cholangitis as well. And rarely, people with primary sclerosing cholangitis develop inflammatory bowel disease only after having a liver transplant.

Risk factors

Factors that may increase the risk of primary sclerosing cholangitis include:

Age. Primary sclerosing cholangitis can occur at any age, but it's most often diagnosed between the ages of 30 and 40.

Sex. Primary sclerosing cholangitis occurs more often in men.

Inflammatory bowel disease. A large proportion of people with primary sclerosing cholangitis also have inflammatory bowel disease.

Geographical location. People with Northern European heritage have a higher risk of primary sclerosing cholangitis.

Symptoms and Diagnosis

Symptoms

The signs and symptoms of PSC change as the disease becomes more advanced. Up to 50% of people may have no symptoms at all at the time of diagnosis. PSC is often found by accident when testing for other conditions. Many people diagnosed with primary sclerosing cholangitis before they have symptoms continue to feel generally well for several years. But there's no reliable way to predict how quickly or slowly the disease will progress for any individual.

The first symptoms to develop tend to be vague. They may include:

• Fatigue.

• Upper right quadrant abdominal pain.

• Itchy skin (pruritus).

Later-stage symptoms may include:

• Swollen abdomen.

• Enlarged liver.

• Enlarged spleen.

• Jaundice.

• Fever.

• Unintended weight loss.

• Chills

• Night sweats

PSC Diagnosis

A diagnosis of PSC begins with a comprehensive physical exam, during which you describe your symptoms and medical history. Other diagnostic procedures include:

- Laboratory tests

- Liver biopsy

- Endoscopic retrograde cholangiopancreatography

- Magnetic resonance cholangiography

Laboratory Tests

Blood tests will be ordered to evaluate your liver function. Patients with PSC almost always have abnormal results. Usually a simple blood test can determine if you have abnormally elevated levels of certain serums.

Liver Biopsy

A liver biopsy is a procedure to remove a piece of liver tissue for laboratory testing. Your doctor inserts a needle through your skin and into your liver to extract a tissue sample.

A liver biopsy can help determine the extent of damage to your liver. The test is used only when the diagnosis of primary sclerosing cholangitis is still uncertain after less-invasive tests.

Endoscopic Retrograde Cholangiopancreatography

An endoscopic retrograde cholangiopancreatography (ERCP) (koh-lan-jee-o-pan-cree-uh-TOG-ruh-fee) is an endoscopic technique that allows visualization of the bile and pancreatic ducts. An endoscope is a thin, flexible, lighted tube that is inserted into your mouth to provide access to your upper gastrointestinal system.

During this procedure:

• A special side-viewing endoscope is used to help place the endoscopic tools into the bile and pancreatic ducts.

• A dye is injected into the ducts to highlight any abnormalities.

• An X-ray is taken to see the ducts

ERCP is the preferred method for visualizing the biliary tree (the network of biliary ducts). Your doctor will find many strictures (narrowing) and dilations (opening), which gives the duct its characteristic beaded appearance.

Magnetic Resonance Cholangiography

Magnetic resonance imaging (MRI) may be useful in detecting blockages. An MRI uses powerful magnetic waves to create a detailed image of the inside of your body. A magnetic resonance cholangiography (MRC) is a specialized MRI used to gather images of the bile ducts.

Complications Associated with PSC

Complications of primary sclerosing cholangitis may include:

• **Liver disease and failure.** Chronic inflammation of the bile ducts throughout your liver can lead to tissue scarring (cirrhosis), liver cell death and, eventually, loss of liver function.

• **Repeated infections**. If scarring of the bile ducts slows or stops the flow of bile out of the liver, you may experience frequent infections in the bile ducts. The risk of infection is particularly high after you've had a surgical procedure to expand a badly scarred bile duct or remove a stone blocking a bile duct.

• **Portal hypertension.** Your portal vein is the major route for blood flowing from your digestive system into your liver. Portal hypertension refers to high blood pressure in this vein.

Portal hypertension can cause fluid from the liver to leak into your abdominal cavity (ascites). It can also divert blood from the portal vein to other veins, causing these veins to become swollen (varices). Varices are weak veins and tend to bleed easily, which can be life-threatening.

• **Thinning bones.** People with primary sclerosing cholangitis may experience thinning bones (osteoporosis). Your doctor may recommend a bone density exam to test for osteoporosis every few years. Calcium and vitamin D supplements may be prescribed to help prevent bone loss.

• **Bile duct cancer.** If you have primary sclerosing cholangitis, you have an increased risk of developing cancer in the bile ducts or gallbladder.

• **Colon cancer.** People with primary sclerosing cholangitis associated with inflammatory bowel disease have an increased risk of colon cancer. If you've been diagnosed with primary sclerosing cholangitis, your doctor may recommend testing for inflammatory bowel disease, even if you have no signs or symptoms, since the risk of colon cancer is elevated if you have both diseases.

Treatment Strategies

Treatments for primary sclerosing cholangitis focus on managing complications and monitoring liver damage. Many medications have been studied in people with primary sclerosing cholangitis, but so far none have been found to slow or reverse the liver damage associated with this disease.

Treatment for itching

• **Bile acid sequestrants.** Medications that bind to bile acids — the substances thought to cause itching in liver disease — are the first line treatment for itching in primary sclerosing cholangitis.

• **Antibiotics.** If you have trouble tolerating a bile acid-binding drug or if it doesn't help, your doctor may prescribe rifampin (Rifadin, Rimactane, others), an antibacterial drug. Exactly how rifampin reduces itching is unknown, but it may block the brain's response to itch-inducing chemicals in your circulation.

• **Antihistamines.** This type of medication may help reduce mild itching caused by primary sclerosing cholangitis. Whether these medications are effective for this condition is unknown.

Antihistamines may worsen the liver disease symptoms of dry eyes and dry mouth. On the other hand, antihistamines can help with sleep if itching keeps you awake.

• **Opioid antagonists.** Itching related to liver disease may also respond to opioid antagonist drugs, such as naltrexone. Like rifampin, these drugs seem to reduce the itch sensation by acting on your brain.

• **Ursodeoxycholic acid (UDCA).** Also known as ursodiol, UDCA is a naturally occurring bile acid that may help relieve itching symptoms caused by liver disease by increasing the absorbability of bile.

Treatment for infections

Bile that backs up in narrowed or blocked ducts causes frequent bacterial infections. To prevent and treat these infections, people with primary sclerosing cholangitis may take repeated courses of antibiotics or continue taking antibiotics for long periods.

Before any procedure that could cause an infection, such as an endoscopic procedure or abdominal surgery, you'll also need to take antibiotics.

Nutrition support

Primary sclerosing cholangitis makes it difficult for your body to absorb certain vitamins. Even though you may eat a healthy diet, you may find that you can't get all the nutrients you need.

Your doctor may recommend vitamin supplements that you take as tablets or that you receive as an infusion through a vein in your arm. If the disease weakens your bones, you may take calcium and vitamin D supplements as well.

Treatment for bile duct blockages

Blockages that occur in your bile ducts may be due to disease progression but can be a sign of cancer of the bile duct. Endoscopic retrograde cholangiopancreatography (ERCP) can help determine the cause, and bile duct blockage can be treated with:

• **Balloon dilation.** This procedure can open blockages in the larger bile ducts outside the liver. In balloon dilation, your doctor runs a slender tube with an inflatable balloon at its tip (balloon catheter) through an endoscope and into a blocked bile duct. Once the balloon catheter is in place, the balloon is inflated.

• **Stent placement.** In this procedure, your doctor uses an endoscope and attached instruments to place a small plastic tube called a stent in a blocked bile duct to hold the duct open.

Liver transplant

A liver transplant is the only treatment known to cure primary sclerosing cholangitis. During a liver transplant, surgeons remove your diseased liver and replace it with a healthy liver from a donor.

A liver transplant is reserved for people with liver failure or other severe complications of primary sclerosing cholangitis. Though uncommon, it's possible for primary sclerosing cholangitis to recur after a liver transplant.

PART II

IMPORTANCE OF DIET IN MANAGING PSC

The liver is the largest gland in the human body, and serves to store nutrients and neutralize harmful substances. The liver plays a very important role in a number of metabolic, both catabolic and anabolic processes, and is therefore called the "central laboratory" of the organism. It is responsible for a large part of the metabolism of carbohydrates, lipids, proteins and other nitrogenous substances. In the liver are also performed processes of detoxification, conjugation and esterification. Metabolic functions are performed in parenchymal cells, hepatocytes, while Kupffer cells are part of the reticuloendothelial system and have the ability to phagocytose. Today, it is already known which subcellular organelles perform some of the above functions.

Metabolic functions involve the normal metabolism of carbohydrates, proteins and fats and have a great influence on the normal circulation of water, vitamins and electrolytes.

Secretory functions include the formation and secretion of bile and its essential components–bile acids, cholesterol and bilirubin. Bile is essential for the breakdown of fats and the absorption of fat-soluble substances including vitamins A, D, E and K.

The liver also serves as a reservoir of blood, vitamins A, D and B12, folic acid and iron as well as a short-term reservoir of small amounts of sugar in the form of glycogen, protein and fat. The liver plays the main role in detoxifying the body from harmful substances.

If liver disease occurs, it can affect all its parts–liver cells, bile ducts, blood and lymph vessels. The liver is damaged by various toxins, drugs, infections, disturbances in the blood supply and other disorders. This creates disorders of liver function that disrupt the metabolic balance of the body, the consequences of which today can be treated with varying degrees of success.

During our lives, we eat tons of food, drink thousands of liters of various beverages, take many different pills, syrups, antibiotics, consume various substances–among them extremely harmful–and all this passes through the liver. Its health is reflected in poor life habits. It will react if we don't eat properly, if we eat in walk, if we cram in large amounts of fatty and baked foods, french fries, chips, donuts, puff pastry, and large amounts of alcohol. Impaired liver function affects the overall health, including the digestive organs that are responsible for quality detoxification of the body. If the liver slows down, the body gradually enters a state of chronic poisoning.

It has been known for a long time that a proper diet can have a beneficial effect on various diseases or mitigate their consequences. Diet therapy has been a part of the process in the treatment of liver disease for a while now. The therapeutic principle is better known as the „liver diet". The liver diet not only mean the replenishment of calories and nutrients, but it significantly affects the course of the disease. Adequate diet therapy, which includes a sufficient number of calories and the proper ratio of essential nutrients with special emphasis on protein content, stems from an understanding of metabolic disorders in the liver.

The diet is not unique to all liver diseases. The main difference is in the amount of protein and the caloric value it contains.

However, for all liver diseases (except for patients with portal encephalopathy), the following recommendations developed by ESPEN in 1997 in order to facilitate the achievement of dietary goals apply.

• Most energy should originate from carbohydrates (60-65%) which are rich in cereals, fruits, vegetables and honey.

• Protein should provide 12-15% (1.0-1.2 g/kg) of total energy per day. The recommended sources of protein are: lean meat, lean cottage cheese, skim milk, eggs and fish.

• The amount of fat should be reduced as much as possible (40-60 grams per day), and it is best to use vegetable fats (e.g. olive oil).

• Vegetables and fruits can be eaten raw or cooked. The salad is prepared with a few drops of olive oil and lemon juice.

• It is desirable to salt the food in moderation, and in case of edema and accumulation of fluid in the abdominal cavity (ascites), an unsalted diet is carried out.

• It is recommended not to prepare dishes with grits, grilled dishes and frying and pouring dishes over heated, cooked or fried fat.

• Food should be taken in more frequent, smaller meals.

• Smoking is not recommended.

• Alcohol is strictly forbidden

In general, here are some key aspects of how diet influences liver health:

1. **Avoidance of Excessive Alcohol**: Alcohol can lead to liver damage, including fatty liver, alcoholic hepatitis, and cirrhosis. Limiting or avoiding alcohol consumption is essential for liver health.

2. **Healthy Weight Management:** Obesity and being overweight increase the risk of non-alcoholic fatty liver disease (NAFLD), which is becoming a leading cause of liver disease worldwide. A balanced diet and regular physical activity are crucial for maintaining a healthy weight.

3. **Balanced Macronutrients:** A diet that includes appropriate amounts of carbohydrates, proteins, and fats is important. Diets too high in refined

carbohydrates or unhealthy fats can contribute to liver fat accumulation.

4. Fiber-Rich Foods: Foods high in fiber, such as fruits, vegetables, and whole grains, can help regulate digestion and reduce the risk of fatty liver disease.

5. Limiting Added Sugars: High intake of sugars, especially fructose, can contribute to liver fat accumulation. Avoiding sugary beverages and processed foods with added sugars is beneficial.

6. Healthy Fats: Unsaturated fats (found in nuts, seeds, avocados, and olive oil) are preferable over saturated fats and trans fats, which can contribute to liver inflammation and damage.

7. Protein Sources: Opt for lean protein sources such as poultry, fish, beans, and legumes. Reducing intake of processed meats and high-fat cuts of meat can help reduce the risk of liver disease.

8. Vitamins and Minerals: Adequate intake of vitamins and minerals, such as vitamin E, vitamin C, and selenium, is important for liver function and protection.

9. Hydration: Drinking enough water is essential for liver health, as it helps the liver detoxify the body and supports overall metabolism.

10. Moderation and Variety: A balanced diet that includes a variety of foods ensures that you get the nutrients your liver needs while minimizing potential harmful effects.

How Diet Can Influence PSC Symptoms

People with primary sclerosing cholangitis (PSC) should eat a healthy, well-balanced diet. Good nutrition is important in all stages of PSC — including cirrhosis — to help the liver work properly and manage complications.

Your doctor can recommend a healthy diet that provides enough calories and nutrients. Your doctor may recommend taking dietary supplements of calcium and vitamin D to help prevent osteoporosis. For low levels of fat-soluble vitamins A, D, E, or K, your doctor may recommend taking supplements of these vitamins. Follow your doctor's instructions on the type and amount of vitamins you should take.

You should avoid eating raw or undercooked shellfish, fish, meat, and unpasteurized milk.

Bacteria or viruses from these foods may cause severe infections in people with liver disease.

Doctors may recommend that people with PSC stop drinking alcohol or, at least, limit their intake. People who have PSC and cirrhosis should completely stop drinking alcohol.

Principles of a PSC-Friendly Diet

Although there is no specific PSC diet, ensuring adequate nutrition along the entire path of a chronic and progressive liver disease is complex, especially where other factors such as diabetes or inflammatory bowel disease co-exist. Below are some principles, however, you should always talk with your doctor or dietician before making any significant dietary changes.

Early Disease

If you are early in your liver disease and still have good liver function, you may not need to adjust your diet. It is still wise to have your micronutrients (see below) checked regularly and add supplements where needed. Maintaining a healthy weight in early PSC will help you manage your disease as it progresses. Sticking to the Australian Healthy Eating pyramid that encourages fruits and vegetables as the highest intake source, followed by grains and then dairy (or dairy alternatives) and meat, with smaller amounts of good fats and sugary treats to be kept to a minimum, should see you manage your diet well.

Advanced Disease

If you are advanced in your PSC it is important that you monitor and try to maintain a healthy weight. Body mass index (BMI) is a score calculated by dividing your weight by your height squared. This gives a rough guide to an appropriate weight for your height but does not allow for other factors such as increased muscle tone (for example, in an athlete), for someone who is retaining additional fluid weight (for example in the liver or heart patient who may have oedema or ascites) or for those whose natural tendency is to be very lean. Some caution should be used in calculating this, and you should not necessarily make it your aim to be within this, but it can give you and your doctor a guide to your healthy weight.

One of the liver's many functions is to store and release glycogen, a chemical in the body that provides us with our energy. As the liver deteriorates in function, the body is forced to rely on other sources of energy, such as protein (eg. Muscle) and fat stores. A high protein diet can provide some protection from muscle loss. The concern of the past was that the high protein may increase the risks of hepatic encephalopathy, but that is no longer considered to be the case.

Another way to minimize muscle breakdown is to consume foods high in energy. You may not be able to tolerate high-fat foods well, so opting for carbohydrate-rich foods such as bread, rice, and pasta will also assist in providing higher energy amounts. Full cream dairy products, or soy products such as soy milk, are also a good nutritional source.

High energy and protein drinks such as Sustagen and Fortsip may also be useful as they are nutritionally complete and provide high nutritional value in quantities more manageable for someone who is not able to tolerate a full diet.

Micronutrients

Micronutrients refer to the vitamins, minerals and trace elements that your body needs in order to function well. There are many of these, but a few are worth a special mention in liver disease.

Fat-soluble vitamins: Vitamins A, D, E and K form the group known as the fat-soluble vitamins. The liver produces bile for these vitamins to be metabolised and used in the body. If the liver is not able to do this adequately nutritional deficiencies occur and require supplementation to reduce the risk of complications. It is important to have these levels checked and supplement them in some form if they are low. However, supplements should only be used in the setting of medical advice and where blood levels have been measured, as they can cause toxicity if they are too high. Supplements may in the form of an oral tablet, injectable into the muscle or via an intravenous infusion. Talk to your doctor about the best form for you.

• Low vitamin A can lead to impaired immunity, issues with the body's ability to produce blood cells, and certain eye disorders including night blindness.

• Low vitamin D can affect bone health, resulting in lower bone density, osteoporosis and potentially some growth issues in children.

• Low Vitamin E can result in muscle weakness and effects on the central nervous system.

• Low vitamin K can lead to poor blood clotting.

Calcium: This is a mineral we have all heard of, and it works alongside Vitamin D to help strengthen bones. A calcium supplement may be required in liver disease due to reduced liver capacity or due to its interaction with some medications.

Magnesium: Another common mineral that requires a supplementation due to poor liver function and interaction with some medications. Lower magnesium can lead to muscle cramping and/or restless leg syndrome. This can be supplemented with an infusion, tablet or even by having an epsom salt bath.

Iron: This can be low in liver disease and often found to be low where there is inflammatory bowel disease (IBD) – particularly at times when the IBD is active. Infusions are available as well as tablets. Low iron can lead to worsening fatigue.

Salt: Even without liver disease many of us eat too much salt to maintain a healthy cardiovascular system. However, in liver disease, the additional issue of fluid build-up, either oedema or ascites, is compounded by too much salt. Avoiding processed foods that contain salt, and not adding salt to your food at the table will help reduce your salt intake. However, for those who have had their colon removed, remember that this is where salt is absorbed, so you may not need to be quite as wary. Check with your specialist or dietician to determine what your salt intake should be.

Specific diets

Especially if you have IBD, you will find resources for a wide variety of diets claiming to be specific to IBD. If these diets have a good nutritional base then it is safe to try them for yourself to see if your symptoms improve. There is no scientifically proven diet for PSC or IBD that will reverse the condition or put it into remission, though some diets are being more heavily studied with promise. Always talk to your specialist or dietician to determine if a specific diet is safe for you to try.

Importance of Fiber and Digestive Health

Fiber feeds "good" gut bacteria

The bacteria that live in the human body outnumber the body's cells 10 to 1. Bacteria live on the skin, in the mouth, and in the nose, but the great majority live in the gut, primarily the large intestine.

Five hundred to 1,000 different species of bacteria live in the intestine, totaling about 38 trillion cells. These gut bacteria are also known as the gut flora.

This is not a bad thing. In fact, there is a mutually beneficial relationship between you and some of the bacteria that live in your digestive system.

You provide food, shelter, and a safe habitat for the bacteria. In return, they take care of some things that the human body cannot do on its own.

Of the many different kinds of bacteria, some are crucial for various aspects of your health, including weight, blood sugar control, immune function, and even brain function.

You may wonder what this has to do with fiber. Just like any other organism, bacteria need to eat to get energy to survive and function.

The problem is that most carbs, proteins, and fats are absorbed into the bloodstream before they make it to the large intestine, leaving little for the gut flora.

This is where fiber comes in. Human cells don't have the enzymes to digest fiber, so it reaches the large intestine relatively unchanged.

However, intestinal bacteria do have the enzymes to digest many of these fibers.

This is the most important reason that (some) dietary fibers are essential for health. They feed the "good" bacteria in the intestine, functioning as prebiotics.

In this way, they promote the growth of "good" gut bacteria, which can have various positive effects on health.

The friendly bacteria produce nutrients for the body, including short-chain fatty acids such as acetate, propionate, and butyrate, of which butyrate appears to be the most important.

These short-chain fatty acids can feed the cells in the colon, leading to reduced gut inflammation and improvements in digestive disorders such as irritable bowel syndrome, Crohn's disease, and ulcerative colitis.

When the bacteria ferment the fiber, they also produce gases. This is why high fiber diets can cause flatulence and stomach discomfort in some people. These side effects usually go away with time as your body adjusts.

Lower Odds of Heart Disease

According to a 2022 BMC Public Health study, a higher fiber intake was associated with a reduced risk for cardiovascular disease (CVD) in a large group of Americans. Researchers don't completely understand how fiber works, but they think that soluble fiber plays a role in decreasing lipid uptake from the intestinal tract, resulting in lower blood levels of cholesterol according to a 2023 Advances in Nutrition review. In addition, experts say that dietary fiber reduces inflammation which can result in CVD in a 2022 JAMA Network Open article.

Some types of fiber can help you lose weight

Certain types of fiber can help you lose weight by reducing your appetite.

In fact, some studies show that increasing dietary fiber can cause weight loss by automatically reducing calorie intake.

Fiber can soak up water in the intestine, slowing the absorption of nutrients and increasing feelings of fullness.

However, this depends on the type of fiber. Some types have no effect on weight, while certain soluble fibers can have a significant effect.

A good example of an effective fiber supplement for weight loss is glucomannan.

Fiber can reduce blood sugar spikes after a high carb meal

High fiber foods tend to have a lower glycemic index than refined carb sources, which have been stripped of most of their fiber.

However, scientists believe that only high viscosity, soluble fibers have this property.

Including these viscous, soluble fibers in your carb-containing meals may cause smaller spikes in blood sugar.

This is important, especially if you're following a high carb diet. In this case, the fiber can reduce the likelihood of the carbs raising your blood sugar to harmful levels.

That said, if you have blood sugar issues, you should consider reducing your carb intake — especially your intake of low fiber, refined carbs such as white flour and added sugar.

Fiber can reduce cholesterol, but the effect isn't huge

Viscous, soluble fiber can also reduce your cholesterol levels.

However, the effect isn't nearly as impressive as you might expect.

A review of 67 controlled studies found that consuming 2–10 grams of soluble fiber per day reduced total cholesterol by only 1.7 mg/dl and LDL (bad) cholesterol by 2.2 mg/dl, on average.

But this also depends on the viscosity of the fiber. Some studies have found impressive reductions in cholesterol with increased fiber intake.

Whether this has any meaningful effects in the long term is unknown, although many observational studies show that people who eat more fiber have a lower risk of heart disease.

Fiber might reduce the risk of colorectal cancer

Colorectal cancer is the third leading cause of cancer deaths in the world.

Many studies have linked a high intake of fiber-rich foods with a reduced risk of colon cancer.

However, whole, high fiber foods like fruits, vegetables, and whole grains contain various other healthy nutrients and antioxidants that may affect cancer risk.

Therefore, it's difficult to isolate the effects of fiber from other factors in healthy, whole-food diets. To date, no strong evidence proves that fiber has cancer-preventive effects.

Yet, since fiber may help keep the colon wall healthy, many scientists believe that fiber plays an important role.

More Regular Bowel Movements

One of the main benefits of increasing fiber intake is reduced constipation.

Fiber is believed to help absorb water, increase the bulk of stool, and speed up the movement of stool through the intestine. However, the evidence is fairly conflicting.

Longer Life

A 2022 review in the Journal of Translational Medicine found that people who ate enough total fiber — which includes soluble and insoluble fibers — had a lower chance of dying early from anything, including cardiovascular disease and cancer. This means that even if you were to get heart disease, cancer or another condition, consuming enough fiber may protect you from dying from it.

Some studies show that increasing fiber can improve symptoms of constipation, but other studies show that removing fiber improves constipation. The effects depend on the type of fiber.

In one study in 63 individuals with chronic constipation, going on a low fiber diet fixed their problem. The individuals who remained on a high fiber diet saw no improvement.

In general, fiber that increases the water content of your stool has a laxative effect, while fiber that adds to the dry mass of stool without increasing its water content may have a constipating effect.

Soluble fibers that form a gel in the digestive tract and are not fermented by gut bacteria are often effective. A good example of a gel-forming fiber is psyllium.

Other types of fiber, such as sorbitol, have a laxative effect by drawing water into the colon. Prunes are a good source of sorbitol.

Choosing the right type of fiber may help your constipation, but taking the wrong supplements can do the opposite.

For this reason, you should consult a healthcare professional before taking fiber supplements for constipation.

All-Natural Detox

Fiber naturally scrubs and promotes the elimination of toxins from your GI tract. Soluble fiber soaks up potentially harmful compounds, such as excess estrogen and unhealthy fats, before they can be absorbed by the body. And because insoluble fiber makes things move along more quickly, it limits the amount of time that chemicals like BPA, mercury and pesticides stay in your system. The faster they go through you, the less chance they have to cause harm.

Strong Bones

Some types of soluble fiber—known as prebiotics—have been shown to contribute to a greater bioavailability of minerals, like calcium, in your colon. The increase in bioavailability supports maintain bone density, according to a 2018 review in the journal Calcified Tissue International. Prebiotics provide food for your beneficial gut bacteria and can be found in certain fruits, vegetables, nuts and whole grains, such as asparagus, bananas, walnuts, onions, legumes, wheat and oats.

PART III

GENERAL DIETARY GUIDELINES FOR PSC

When it comes to managing primary sclerosing cholangitis (PSC), a healthy diet plays a crucial role in supporting liver health and reducing inflammation. Incorporating specific foods that are beneficial for individuals with PSC can provide essential nutrients and compounds that promote overall well-being. Here are some examples of foods rich in these nutrients and suggestions for incorporating them into your diet:

1. Fatty Fish: Fatty fish like salmon, mackerel, and sardines are excellent sources of omega-3 fatty acids. These healthy fats have anti-inflammatory properties and can help reduce liver inflammation. Aim to include fatty fish in your diet at least twice a week.

2. Colorful Fruits and Vegetables: Opt for a variety of colorful fruits and vegetables, as they are packed with antioxidants and phytochemicals that support liver health. Include berries, leafy greens, bell peppers, carrots, and tomatoes in your meals to reap their benefits.

3. Whole Grains: Replace refined grains with whole grains like brown rice, quinoa, and whole wheat bread. These complex carbohydrates provide fiber, vitamins, and minerals that aid digestion and promote a healthy gut, which is essential for individuals with PSC.

4. Healthy Fats: Incorporate healthy fats into your diet, such as avocados, nuts, and olive oil. These fats are rich in monounsaturated and polyunsaturated fats, which can help reduce inflammation and support liver function.

5. Herbal Teas: Certain herbal teas like green tea, dandelion root tea, and milk thistle tea have been associated with liver health benefits. These teas contain antioxidants and compounds that may help protect the liver from damage.

Remember to consult with your healthcare provider or a registered dietitian before making any significant changes to your diet. They can provide personalized recommendations based on your specific needs and medical condition. By incorporating these foods into your diet, you can take an active role in supporting your liver health and managing primary sclerosing cholangitis.

Foods to Limit or Avoid

When following a primary sclerosing cholangitis (PSC) diet, it is important to avoid or limit certain foods that can worsen symptoms or contribute to liver damage. Here are some foods that should be avoided:

1. Fatty Foods: Foods high in saturated and trans fats, such as fried foods, fatty cuts of meat, full-fat dairy products, and processed snacks, should be avoided. These foods can increase inflammation and put extra strain on the liver.

2. Alcohol: Alcohol is known to cause liver damage and should be completely avoided if you have PSC. It can worsen symptoms and lead to further complications.

3. High Sodium Foods: Foods high in sodium, such as processed meats, canned soups, and fast food, should be limited. High sodium intake can contribute to fluid retention and increase blood pressure.

4. Spicy Foods: Spicy foods can irritate the digestive system and worsen symptoms like abdominal pain and diarrhea. It is best to avoid or limit spicy foods.

5. Refined Sugars: Foods high in refined sugars, such as sugary drinks, candies, and desserts, should be limited. These foods can contribute to weight gain and inflammation.

Instead of these restricted foods, you can opt for healthier alternatives:

1. Lean Proteins: Choose lean sources of protein such as skinless poultry, fish, legumes, and tofu.

These provide essential nutrients without the added fat.

2. Whole Grains: Replace refined grains with whole grains like brown rice, quinoa, and whole wheat bread. These are higher in fiber and provide more nutrients.

3. Fresh Fruits and Vegetables: Include a variety of fresh fruits and vegetables in your diet. They are rich in antioxidants and fiber, which can help reduce inflammation.

4. Healthy Fats: Include sources of healthy fats like avocados, nuts, and olive oil in moderation. These can provide essential nutrients without putting strain on the liver.

5. Low Sodium Options: Opt for low sodium alternatives or prepare meals at home using fresh ingredients to control your sodium intake.

By avoiding or limiting these foods and choosing healthier options, you can support your liver health and manage symptoms of primary sclerosing cholangitis.

Meal Planning Tips

When following a primary sclerosing cholangitis (PSC) diet, meal planning becomes essential to ensure you are getting the right nutrients while avoiding foods that may worsen your symptoms. Here are some practical tips and strategies to help you with your meal planning:

1. **Portion Control:** It is important to be mindful of portion sizes to prevent overeating and to maintain a healthy weight. Use measuring cups or

a food scale to accurately measure your food portions.

2. **Balanced Meals**: Aim to include a variety of food groups in each meal to ensure you are getting a balanced intake of nutrients. Include lean proteins, such as chicken, fish, or tofu, along with whole grains, fruits, vegetables, and healthy fats.

3. **Regular Eating Patterns:** Establishing regular eating patterns can help regulate your digestion and prevent symptoms associated with PSC. Try to eat at the same times each day and avoid skipping meals.

Sample Meal Plan:

- Breakfast: Oatmeal topped with fresh berries and a tablespoon of almond butter.

- Snack: Greek yogurt with sliced cucumbers.

 - Lunch: Grilled chicken breast with quinoa and steamed vegetables.

- Snack: Apple slices with a handful of almonds.

 - Dinner: Baked salmon with roasted sweet potatoes and a side salad.

Recipe Ideas:

- Quinoa Salad with Roasted Vegetables: Toss cooked quinoa with roasted bell peppers, zucchini, and cherry tomatoes. Drizzle with olive oil and lemon juice.

- Grilled Chicken and Vegetable Skewers: Thread marinated chicken breast, bell peppers, onions, and cherry tomatoes onto skewers. Grill until chicken is cooked through.

- Baked Salmon with Lemon and Dill: Place salmon fillets on a baking sheet, drizzle with lemon juice, sprinkle with fresh dill, and bake until fish is flaky.

By following these meal planning tips, you can support a healthy PSC diet and improve your overall well-being.

Making Healthy Food Choices

When it comes to managing primary sclerosing cholangitis (PSC), making healthy food choices is crucial for maintaining overall well-being. Whether you are dining out or grocery shopping, here are some tips to help you navigate your options and maintain a nutritious diet.

1. Label Reading: When grocery shopping, it's important to read food labels carefully. Look for products that are low in saturated fats, trans fats, and cholesterol. Pay attention to the sodium content as well, as excessive sodium intake can worsen symptoms of PSC. Opt for foods that are high in fiber, such as whole grains, fruits, and vegetables.

2. Identifying Hidden Ingredients: Some foods may contain hidden ingredients that can trigger symptoms or worsen liver function. For example, certain sauces, dressings, and marinades may contain high amounts of fat, sugar, or artificial additives. Be mindful of these hidden ingredients and choose options that are lower in fat and sugar.

3. Navigating Restaurant Menus: Eating out can be challenging when you have specific dietary restrictions. However, many restaurants now offer healthier options on their menus. Look for dishes that are grilled, steamed, or baked instead of fried. Choose lean protein sources like fish, chicken, or tofu. Ask for sauces and dressings on the side to control the amount you consume.

4. Tips for Enjoying Meals outside the Home: While it's important to make healthy choices, it's also essential to enjoy your meals outside the home. Here are some tips to help you strike a balance:

- Practice portion control: Restaurants often serve larger portions, so consider sharing a meal or taking leftovers home. - Choose water or unsweetened beverages instead of sugary drinks. - Opt for fresh fruits or yogurt for dessert instead of high-sugar options. - Be mindful of your overall calorie intake and balance it with physical activity.

By being mindful of your food choices, reading labels, and making informed decisions, you can maintain a nutritious diet while still enjoying meals outside the home.

PART I

DELICIOUSLY SIMPLE RECIPES
YOU MUST TRY!

BREAKFAST RECIPES FOR PSC

Roasted stone fruits with vanilla

Ingredients

- 175g golden caster sugar

- 1 vanilla pod, split in two

- 5 cardamom pods

- zest and juice 1 lime

- 6 apricots, halved and stoned

- 3 peaches, quartered and stoned

- 3 nectarines, quartered and stoned

Directions

- STEP 1

Heat oven to 220C/fan 200C/gas 8. Tip the sugar, vanilla pod, cardamom, lime zest and juice into a food processor, then blitz until blended, or mash together using a pestle and mortar. Tip the fruit into a shallow baking dish, then toss in the sludgy sugar.

• STEP 2

Roast for 20 mins until the fruits have softened, but not collapsed and the sugar and fruit juices have made a sticky sauce. Any leftovers will keep in the fridge for up to 2 days.

Banana, clementine & mango smoothie

Ingredients

• about 24 juicy clementines, plus an extra one for decoration

* 2 small, very ripe and juicy mangoes

* 2 ripe bananas

* 500g tub whole milk or low-fat yogurt

* handful of ice cubes (optional)

Directions

* STEP 1

Halve the clementines and squeeze out the juice –
you should have about 600ml/1 pint. (This can be
done the night before.) Peel the mangoes, slice the
fruit away from the stone in the centre, then chop
the flesh into rough pieces. Peel and slice the
bananas.

* STEP 2

Put the clementine juice, mango flesh, bananas,
yogurt and ice cubes into a liquidiser and blend

until smooth. Pour into six glasses and serve. (You might need to make this in two batches, depending on the size of your liquidiser.) If you don't add ice cubes, chill in the fridge until ready to serve.

Hash browns with gruyère & pancetta

Ingredients

- 800g Maris Piper or King Edward potatoes

- 1 ½ tbsp olive oil

- 1 small onion, finely diced

- 2 garlic cloves

- 75g pancetta, diced

- 50g gruyère, grated

- small pack parsley, chopped

• 2 large eggs, lightly beaten

• roasted cherry tomatoes and mushrooms, to serve (optional)

Directions

• STEP 1

Peel the potatoes, cut them into large chunks and put them in a saucepan of cold salted water. Bring to the boil and simmer for 15 mins until just cooked (do not overcook or the potatoes will absorb too much water).

• STEP 2

Meanwhile, heat 1/2 tbsp of the olive oil in a small pan. Add the onion, garlic and a pinch of salt, then cover and cook over a low heat for 15-20 mins until the onion is soft and starting to caramelise. If the onion starts to catch, add a splash of cold water.

Remove the onion and garlic, then fry the pancetta in the same pan until the fat has melted and the pancetta is crisp.

• STEP 3

Drain the potatoes and allow to steam-dry. Once cool enough to handle, chop the potatoes into 1cm dice and mix in a bowl with the pancetta, gruyère, parsley, beaten eggs, onion and garlic. Season generously with black pepper.

• STEP 4

Heat 1 tbsp of the oil in a large non-stick frying pan. Gently tip in the potato mixture and press down with the back of a large spoon. Fry over a medium heat for 15 mins until the bottom is golden brown. Tip the hash brown onto a plate, then slide back into the pan, cooked-side up. Cook for another 15 mins until golden and hot. Serve with roasted tomatoes and mushrooms, if you like.

Mango & passion fruit smoothie

Ingredients

- 400g/14oz peeled and chopped ripe mango

- 2 x 125g pots fat-free mango yogurt

- 250ml skimmed milk

- juice 1 lime

- 4 passion fruits, halved

Directions

- STEP 1

Whizz the mango, yogurt and milk together in a blender until smooth. Stir in the lime juice, then pour into 4 glasses. Scoop the pulp of a passion fruit into each one, and swirl before serving.

Oven-baked egg & chips

Ingredients

- 2 medium baking potatoes, cut into chunky wedges

- 2 tbsp olive oil

- 1 tsp smoked paprika

- 2 tomatoes, halved

- 2 eggs

Directions

- STEP 1

Heat oven to 190C/170C fan/gas 5. Tip the potato wedges into a roasting tin. Drizzle over the oil and sprinkle over the paprika. Season and mix well to coat the potatoes. Roast for 25 mins, turning halfway through, until almost tender.

- STEP 2

Nestle the tomatoes, cut-side up, amongst the potatoes. Make 2 spaces in the tin and crack an egg into each one. Return to the oven for 6-8 mins until the eggs are just set.

Cherry-Berry Smoothie Bowl

Ingredients

- 1 cup unsweetened tart cherry juice, chilled

- 1 cup packed baby spinach

- 3/4 cup plain 2% reduced-fat strained yogurt

- 1 ripe avocado, peeled and pitted

- 3/4 cup unsweetened frozen mixed berries

- 2 tablespoons chia seeds

- 1 1/4 cups fresh mixed berries

Directions

1. Place juice, spinach, yogurt, avocado and frozen berries in a blender; process until smooth. Divide between 2 bowls and top with chia seeds and fresh berries. Serve immediately.

Spanakopita Breakfast Sandwiches

Ingredients

- 2 tablespoons extra-virgin olive oil, divided

- 4 large eggs

- ¼ cup finely chopped onion

- 1 (5 ounce) package baby spinach

- 3 cups arugula

- 1 tablespoon chopped fresh dill

- ½ teaspoon garlic powder

- ¼ teaspoon ground pepper

- ⅛ teaspoon salt

- 4 whole-wheat English muffins, split and toasted

- 4 tablespoons crumbled feta cheese

Directions

1. Heat 1 tablespoon oil in a large skillet over medium heat. Break eggs, one at a time, into the pan. Cook until the whites are set but the yolks are still runny, 1 to 2 minutes. Break the yolks with a spatula. Flip the eggs and cook until just done, about 1 minute more. Transfer to a plate and cover to keep warm.

2. Add the remaining 1 tablespoon oil and onion to the pan. Cook, stirring often, until softened, about 1 minute. Add spinach and arugula in batches and cook, stirring, until wilted, about 4 minutes. Add dill, garlic powder, pepper and salt; cook, stirring, for 1 minute more.

3. To assemble sandwiches, place the eggs on the bottom halves of the English muffins. Top each with ¼ cup of the spinach mixture, then sprinkle with 1 tablespoon feta (reserve excess spinach

mixture for another use). Serve topped with the remaining muffin halves.

Frittata

Ingredients

- 8 large eggs

- ¼ cup half-and-half

- ¼ teaspoon salt, divided

- ⅛ teaspoon ground pepper

- 2 tablespoons extra-virgin olive oil

- ¾ cup chopped onion (such as white, yellow or sweet) or shallot

- 1 teaspoon grated garlic

- ⅓ cup chopped bell peppers (yellow, red or orange)

- ¼ cup finely chopped mushrooms, broccoli or cauliflower

- 1 cup chopped leafy greens (such as kale or spinach)

- ¼ cup chopped fresh herbs (such as basil, parsley, dill or chives), plus more for garnish

- ½ cup shredded sharp Cheddar cheese

- ¼ cup grated low-moisture cheese (such as Parmesan or cotija)

- ⅛ teaspoon crushed red pepper

Directions

1. Preheat oven to 400°F. Whisk eggs, half-and-half, 1/8 teaspoon salt and pepper in a medium bowl until thoroughly blended and smooth.

2. Heat oil in a 10-inch cast-iron skillet over medium-high heat. Add onion (or shallot), garlic and the remaining 1/8 teaspoon salt; cook, stirring occasionally, until the onion is mostly translucent, about 2 minutes. Add peppers and mushrooms (or broccoli or cauliflower); cook, stirring occasionally, until softened, about 2 minutes. Add leafy greens and herbs; cook, stirring occasionally, until the greens are bright green, wilted and starting to dry out around the edges, about 2 minutes.

3. Reduce heat to low. Pour in the egg mixture. Add cheeses, using a silicone spatula or fork to carefully arrange the mixture evenly; sprinkle with crushed red pepper. Transfer the skillet to the

oven; bake until the eggs are set in the center, 10 to 15 minutes. Garnish with additional fresh herbs, if desired.

High-Fiber Matcha Green Smoothie Bowl

Ingredients

- 1/2 cup frozen banana slices

- 1/2 cup frozen sliced peaches

- 1/2 cup spinach

- 1/2 cup unsweetened almond milk

- 5 tablespoons sliced almonds, divided

- 1 1/2 teaspoons matcha tea powder

- 1 teaspoon pure maple syrup

• 1/2 ripe kiwi, sliced

Directions

1. Place banana, peaches, spinach, almond milk, 3 tablespoons almonds, matcha and maple syrup in a blender; process until smooth. Pour into a bowl and top with kiwi and the remaining 2 tablespoons almonds. Serve immediately.

Yasai-To-Tofu-no-Misoshiru (Hearty Miso Soup with Vegetables & Tofu)

Ingredients

Dashi

• 5 ½ cups water

• 1 4-inch square kombu

• 3 cups (20 grams) bonito flakes

Miso Soup

- 2 tablespoons light sesame oil

- ½ medium onion, halved and sliced 1/4 inch thick

- 2 medium carrots, sliced 1/4 inch thick

- 6 ounces sweet potato, preferably satsuma, diced (1/4-inch)

- 4 ounces daikon, peeled, quartered and sliced 1/4 inch thick

- 3 ounces shiitake mushrooms, stems removed, sliced 1/4 inch thick

- 4 tablespoons red and/or white miso

- 8 ounces soft or medium-firm tofu, cut into 1/4-inch cubes

- 2 scallions, sliced

- ½ teaspoon grated lemon zest

- Shichimi togarashi for garnish

Directions

1. To prepare dashi: Heat water and kombu in a large pot over medium heat until bubbles begin to form around the kombu, 5 to 10 minutes. Remove the kombu, continue cooking until the water comes to a boil, then remove from heat. Add bonito flakes and let stand for 2 minutes. Strain the dashi through a fine-mesh sieve into a large glass measuring cup or heatproof bowl. (Do not press the bonito flakes while straining as it will cloud the dashi.) You should have 5 cups.

2. To prepare miso soup: Heat oil in a large saucepan over medium heat. Add onion and cook,

stirring occasionally, until soft, about 5 minutes. Add carrots, sweet potato, daikon and shiitakes. Cook, stirring occasionally, until the vegetables start to soften, about 5 minutes. Add 4 3/4 cups of the dashi and bring to a boil over medium-high heat. Reduce heat to maintain a simmer and cook until the vegetables are soft, about 6 minutes.

3. Pour the remaining 1/4 cup dashi into a small bowl and whisk in miso. Add the miso mixture and tofu to the soup and stir. Serve the miso soup topped with scallions and lemon zest and garnished with shichimi, if desired.

Spinach, Mushroom & Egg Casserole

Ingredients

- 2 tablespoons extra-virgin olive oil

• 1 pound cremini mushrooms, trimmed and sliced

• 5 medium cloves garlic, finely chopped

• 2 teaspoons dry mustard

• 1 teaspoon onion powder

• 1 teaspoon salt

• 5 ounces baby spinach

• 12 large eggs

• ¾ cup half-and-half

• 1 ½ cups shredded Gruyère cheese, preferably cave-aged (see Tip), divided

• 2 teaspoons fresh thyme leaves

Directions

1. Preheat oven to 375°F. Coat a 9-by-13-inch baking dish with cooking spray. Heat oil in a large skillet over medium-high heat. Add mushrooms in an even layer; cook, undisturbed, until starting to brown, 5 to 6 minutes. Stir and continue to cook, undisturbed, until golden brown on the bottom, about 3 minutes. Stir and continue to cook, stirring occasionally, until the mushrooms are browned all over and the liquid has evaporated, about 3 minutes. Add garlic, dry mustard, onion powder and salt; cook, stirring constantly, until fragrant, about 1 minute. Add spinach and cook, stirring constantly, until the spinach wilts, 1 to 2 minutes. Set aside to cool slightly, about 10 minutes.

2. Crack eggs into a large bowl and whisk until completely smooth. Add half-and-half and whisk until combined. Reserve 1/2 cup of the vegetable mixture; scatter the remaining mixture in the prepared baking dish. Sprinkle evenly with 3/4

cup Gruyère. Pour the egg mixture over the top. Sprinkle evenly with the remaining 3/4 cup Gruyère and the reserved 1/2 cup vegetable mixture. Bake until puffed, golden brown and just set, 30 to 35 minutes. Let cool slightly, about 10 minutes. Sprinkle with thyme before serving.

Tip

Cave-aged Gruyère is aged for at least a year in caves that provide the perfect environment for aging which intensifies the flavor and hardens the texture of the cheese. Look for it in well-stocked supermarkets, specialty cheese shops or online. While cave-aged Gruyère adds depth of flavor to this recipe, regular Gruyère will work well too.

Almond crêpes with avocado & nectarines

Ingredients

- 2 large eggs

- 3 tbsp ground almonds

- 2 tsp rapeseed oil

- 1 avocado, halved, stoned and flesh lightly crushed

- 2 ripe nectarines, stoned and sliced

- seeds from 1/2 pomegranate

- ½ lime, cut into 2 wedges, for squeezing over

Instructions

- STEP 1

Beat one egg and 1 1 /2 tbsp of the almonds in a small bowl with 1 tbsp water. Heat 1 tsp oil in a large non-stick frying pan over a medium heat and pour in the egg mixture, swirling the pan to evenly cover the base. Cook until the mixture sets and turns golden on the underside, about 2 mins. (There is no need to flip it over.) Turn it out onto a plate and make another one with 1 tbsp water, the remaining egg, oil and almonds.

• STEP 2

Top each crêpe with the avocado, nectarines and pomegranate, and squeeze over the lime at the table.

Millet porridge with almond milk & berry compote

Ingredients

• 340g millet

• 1 litre unsweetened fortified almond milk, plus extra to serve

- few mint leaves, to serve

For the compote

- 90g pitted dates, finely chopped

- 500g frozen mixed fruit (ours was a mixed bag of berries, cherries, currants and strawberries)

- 1 cinnamon stick

Instructions

- STEP 1

For the compote, put the dates in a pan with 150ml water, bring to the boil and stir well so they break down. Tip in the frozen fruit and cinnamon stick and cook over a medium heat, stirring every now and then for a couple of minutes. Don't worry about fully thawing larger fruits, as they will defrost in the residual heat and retain their shape in the compote (if you have large strawberries in the mix, you can halve these as they soften). Leave to cool. Will then keep chilled for up to four days.

• STEP 2

Rinse the millet in a sieve, then tip into a deep, heavy-based saucepan and pour in the almond milk and 350ml water. Put over a low heat and once bubbling, leave to simmer for 10-12 mins, stirring frequently until the millet grains are tender, but nutty.

Serve the porridge with the compote. Add a little extra almond milk to serve with a few mint leaves scattered over.

Berry omelette

Ingredients

* 1 large egg

* 1 tbsp skimmed milk

* 3 pinches of cinnamon

* ½ tsp rapeseed oil

* 100g cottage cheese

* 175g chopped strawberry, blueberries and raspberries

Instructions

* STEP 1

Beat egg with milk and cinnamon. Heat oil in a 20cm non-stick frying pan and pour in the egg mixture, swirling to evenly cover the base. Cook for a few mins until set and golden underneath. There's no need to flip it over.

• STEP 2

Place on a plate, spread over cheese, then scatter with berries. Roll up and serve.

Creamy smoked haddock & saffron kedgeree

Ingredients

• 300g basmati rice

• 50g butter

• 3 hard-boiled eggs, shelled and halved

• 200ml double cream

• 500g naturally smoked haddock, skin removed

• 100ml white wine

• 1tsp cayenne pepper

- pinch saffron strands

- 1 tbsp mild curry powder

- freshly grated nutmeg

- small handful flat-leaf parsley, chopped

- 1 lemon, cut into wedges, to serve

Instructions

- STEP 1

Cook basmati rice, leave to cool. Heat oven to 160C/140C fan/gas 3. Grease a large ovenproof dish with some of the butter. Push the egg yolks through a sieve and roughly chop the whites.

- STEP 2

Gently heat the cream in a frying pan until just below boiling point, then add the fish. Cover and poach for 4 mins. Place the wine in a pan with the saffron and warm to infuse. In a large bowl, mix together the rice, cayenne, curry powder, nutmeg, seasoning, chopped egg whites and saffron-infused wine. Lift the fish out of the cream and flake into the bowl – removing any bones as you find them. Scrape in the cream and gently mix together once more.

• STEP 3

Tip everything into the buttered dish and dot the top with the remaining butter. Bake to heat through for 20 mins, then serve scattered with the parsley and sieved egg yolk, with lemon wedges on the side.

Kale & salmon kedgeree

Ingredients

- 300g brown rice

- 2 salmon fillets (about 280g)

- 4 eggs

- 1 tbsp vegetable oil

- 1 onion, finely chopped

- 100g curly kale, stalks removed, roughly chopped

- 1 garlic clove, crushed

- 1 tbsp curry powder

- 1 tsp turmeric

- zest and juice 1 lemon

Instructions

- STEP 1

Cook the rice following pack instructions. Meanwhile, season the salmon and steam over a pan of simmering water for 8 mins or until just cooked. Keep the pan of water on the heat, add the eggs and boil for 6 mins, then run under cold water.

• STEP 2

Heat the oil in a large frying pan or wok, add the onion and cook for 5 mins. Throw in the kale and cook, stirring, for 5 mins. Add the garlic, curry powder, turmeric and rice, season and stir until heated through.

• STEP 3

Peel and quarter the eggs. Flake the salmon and gently fold through the rice, then divide between plates and top with the eggs. Sprinkle over the lemon zest and squeeze over a little juice before serving.

Cured salmon

Ingredients

- 1 tbsp cracked black pepper

- 75g muscovado sugar

- 60g sea salt flakes

- 1 filleted side of very fresh salmon (about 800g), skin on

For the dill & lemon cream cheese

- 200g full-fat cream cheese, at room temperature

- small bunch of dill, finely chopped

- ½ unwaxed lemon, zested and juiced, plus extra wedges to serve

For the pickle

- 1 small cucumber

- 1 small red onion, finely sliced

- pinch of caster sugar

- 3 tbsp white wine vinegar

To serve

- selection of toasted bagels

- sliced rye bread

- small pot of salmon caviar

- caper berries or capers, drained

Instructions

• STEP 1

Up to four days but at least two days before serving the salmon, mix the pepper, sugar and salt together. Pat the salmon dry with kitchen paper and run your hands over the flesh to find any stray bones – use tweezers to pull these out, if needed. Lay the salmon in a dish, skin-side down, and pack the salt mix over the flesh. Cover the fish with a board or tray weighed down with a few heavy cans or jars. Transfer to the fridge for at least two days or up to four, turning the fillet about every 12 hrs.

• STEP 2

To make the dill cream cheese, beat all of the Ingredients together and set aside. This can be made up to a day ahead and chilled.

• STEP 3

To make the pickle, cut the cucumber in half lengthways, scoop out the seeds using a spoon, and slice into thin half-moons. Toss the cucumber with the red onion and a generous pinch of salt in a colander, then set aside for 30 mins to soften. Transfer the vegetables to a bowl or jar and top up with the sugar and vinegar. Can be eaten immediately or made up to two days ahead and chilled.

• STEP 4

Lift the salmon out of the curing mixture and wipe off any excess seasoning using kitchen paper. Put the fish on a large serving board and carve into thin slices. Serve with the bagels and rye bread, dill & lemon cream cheese, the pickle, salmon caviar, capers and lemon wedges.

LUNCH RECIPES FOR PSC

Tomato, watermelon & feta salad with mint dressing

Ingredients

- 2 tbsp olive oil

- 1 tbsp red wine vinegar

- ¼ tsp chilli flakes

- 2 tbsp chopped mint

- 4 tomatoes, chopped

- 500g/1lb 2oz watermelon, cut into chunks

- 200g pack feta cheese, crumbled

Instructions

- STEP 1

Make the dressing by mixing the oil, vinegar, chilli flakes and mint with some seasoning.

- STEP 2

Put the tomatoes and watermelon in a bowl. Pour over the dressing and leave to stand for 10 mins to allow the fruit to get really juicy. Gently stir through the feta, then serve.

Roasted summer vegetable casserole

Ingredients

- 3 tbsp olive oil

- 1 garlic bulb, halved through the middle

- 2 large courgettes, thickly sliced

- 1 large red onion, sliced

- 1 aubergine, halved and sliced on the diagonal

- 2 large tomatoes, quartered

- 200g new potatoes, scrubbed and halved

- 1 red pepper, deseeded and cut into chunky pieces

- 400g can chopped tomatoes

- 0.5 small pack parsley, chopped

Instructions

- STEP 1

Heat oven to 200C/180C fan/gas 6 and put the oil in a roasting tin. Tip in the garlic and all the fresh veg, then toss with your hands to coat in the oil. Season well and roast for 45 mins.

• STEP 2

Remove the garlic from the roasting tin and squeeze out the softened cloves all over the veg, stirring to evenly distribute. In a medium pan, simmer the chopped tomatoes until bubbling, season well and stir through the roasted veg in the tin. Scatter over the parsley and serve.

Bean & quinoa salad with orange

Ingredients

• 120g quinoa

• 320g celery, strings removed if tough, sliced

• 320g frozen soya beans

• 2 tbsp extra virgin olive oil

• 3 tbsp apple cider vinegar

- 8 spring onions, trimmed and thinly sliced

- 30g flat-leaf parsley, chopped

- 4 tbsp chopped mint (optional)

- 4 small oranges, peeled and segmented

- 120g feta, crumbled

Instructions

- STEP 1

Tip the quinoa and celery into a pan and cover with plenty of water. Bring to the boil, then reduce the heat and simmer for 10 mins. Add the soya beans, bring back to the boil and cook for 7 mins more. Drain well, tip into a bowl and set aside.

- STEP 2

Add the oil, vinegar and spring onions, and leave to cool slightly before stirring in the parsley and mint. Serve two portions topped with half the segmented oranges and half the feta crumbled over. Chill the remaining salad for another day, then segment the remaining oranges and crumble over the feta just before serving. Will keep chilled in an airtight container for up to three days.

Tuna, avocado & pea salad in Baby Gem lettuce wraps

Ingredients

• 1 ½ tbsp low-fat natural yogurt

• 85g canned tuna chunks (in spring water), drained

• 50g cooked and cooled rice (use leftover from Prawn, butternut & mango curry dinner if made - see 'goes well with', right)

• 85g frozen pea, cooked, then refreshed in cold water

• ½ red pepper, chopped

• 1 avocado, stoned, peeled and cut into chunks

• zest and juice 1 lime

• small pack coriander, chopped

• 1 large Baby Gem lettuce, or other crisp lettuce, such as cos

Instructions

• STEP 1

Combine all the Ingredients except the lettuce in a bowl, season, then chill until ready to eat. Spoon the tuna mix on top of the lettuce leaves, wrap up and enjoy.

Watermelon, prawn & avocado salad

Ingredients

• 1 small red onion, finely chopped

• 1 fat garlic clove, crushed

• 1 small red chilli, finely chopped

• juice 1 lime

• 1 tbsp rice or white wine vinegar

• 1 tsp caster sugar

• watermelon wedge, deseeded and diced

- 1 avocado, diced

- small bunch coriander leaves, chopped

- 200g cooked tiger prawns, defrosted if frozen

Instructions

- STEP 1

Put the onion in a medium bowl with the garlic, chilli, lime juice, vinegar, sugar and some seasoning. Leave to marinate for 10 mins.

- STEP 2

Add the watermelon, avocado, coriander and prawns, then toss gently to serve.

Smoked mackerel & beetroot salad with creamy horseradish dressing

Ingredients

• 6-10 beetroots (depending on size)

• 140g puy lentils, cooked

• bunch spring onions (about 8), sliced on an angle

• 1 eating apple, core removed, thinly sliced (squeeze a little lemon juice over to prevent them turning brown)

• 1 small radicchio, leaves separated and torn into bite-sized chunks

• 1 pack smoked mackerel (approx 250g), skin and any bones removed, flaked into chunky pieces

For the horseradish dressing

- zest and juice 1 lemon

- 150ml pot soured cream

- 2 tbsp creamed horseradish

Instructions

- STEP 1

Heat oven to 200C/180C fan/gas 6. Place the unpeeled beetroots on a baking tray and roast for 35-50 mins, depending on their size. Give them a gentle squeeze after 35 mins – if they feel tender and are a little shrivelled, they are done; if not, continue cooking. Remove from the oven and set aside to cool.

- STEP 2

Using a small sharp knife, carefully peel the beetroots, then cut into wedges (wear plastic gloves to prevent them staining your hands). Mix the dressing Ingredients in a small bowl. Put the lentils, spring onions, apple, radicchio and mackerel in a large bowl, add half the dressing and toss everything together. Pile the Ingredients onto a serving platter, layering with the beetroots as you do. Serve with the remaining dressing on the side.

BBQ mackerel

Ingredients

- 3 tbsp extra-virgin olive oil

- 4 small whole mackerel, gutted and cleaned

For the drizzle

- 1 large red chilli, deseeded and finely chopped

- 1 small garlic clove, finely chopped

- small knob fresh root ginger, finely chopped

- 2 tsp honey

- 2 limes, zested and juiced

- 1 tsp sesame oil

- 1 tsp Thai fish sauce

Directions

- STEP 1

Light the barbecue and allow the flames to die down until the ashes have gone white with heat. Make the drizzle by whisking 2 tbsp olive oil and all the other Ingredients together in a small bowl, adjusting the ratio of honey and lime to make a sharp sweetness. Season to taste.

* STEP 2

Score each side of the mackerel about 6 times, not quite through to the bone. Brush the fish with the remaining oil and season lightly. Barbecue the mackerel for 5-6 mins on each side until the fish is charred and the eyes have turned white. Spoon the drizzle over the fish and allow to stand for 2-3 mins before serving.

Korean fishcakes with fried eggs & spicy salsa

Ingredients

For the fishcakes

* 4 x loch trout or rainbow trout fillets, skinned and cut into 1cm/ 1/2in pieces (about 450g/1lb fish)

- 2 tsp finely grated ginger

- 1 fat garlic clove, crushed

- 1 tsp light soy sauce

- bunch spring onions, thinly sliced

- 1 large egg white, beaten until frothy

- 2 tbsp rice flour

- 2 ½ tbsp vegetable oil, for frying

For the salad

- 1 pointed or small white cabbage, cored and finely shredded (about 350g/12oz)

- 100g radishes, thinly sliced

- 2 tbsp Chinese rice vinegar

- 1 tbsp sesame oil, plus 2 tsp to serve

- 1 tsp gochujang, plus 2 top to serve (see tip)

- 1 tsp golden caster sugar

- 1 garlic clove, crushed

- 2 tsp light soy sauce

- 4 medium eggs

- 1 tbsp sesame seeds, toasted

- 1 red chilli, finely sliced, to serve (optional)

Directions

- STEP 1

For the fishcakes, mix the fish with the ginger, garlic, soy and half the spring onions. Stir in the egg white and rice flour.

- STEP 2

Toss the cabbage and radishes with the vinegar, 1 tbsp sesame oil, 1 tsp gochujang, the sugar and garlic. Set aside. Stir together the remaining sesame oil, gochujang and the soy sauce to make a drizzling sauce for later.

• STEP 3

Heat 1 tbsp oil in a large, non-stick frying pan. Split the fish mixture into eight, then spoon four into the pan, pressing the mix to make cakes about 8cm across. Fry for 2 mins each side until just cooked through and golden. Add another 1 tbsp oil to the pan and repeat with the remaining fish. Keep warm in a low oven.

• STEP 4

Add the remaining oil to the pan. Fry the eggs for 2-3 mins until crisp but with a runny yolk. Serve the fishcakes with the cabbage, and top with the egg and sesame seeds. Scatter with the rest of the spring onions, red chilli (if using) and some of the chilli sesame drizzle.

Classic lasagne

Ingredients

- 2 olive oil, plus extra for the dish

- 750g lean beef mince

- 90g pack prosciutto

- 800g passata or half our basic tomato sauce

- 200ml hot beef stock

- nutmeg

- 300g fresh lasagne sheets

• white sauce (find a recipe in the Directions, or use shop-bought)

• 125g ball mozzarella, torn into thin strips

Directions

• STEP 1

To make the meat sauce, heat 2 tbsp olive oil in a frying pan and cook 750g lean beef mince in two batches for about 10 mins until browned all over.

• STEP 2

Finely chop 4 slices of prosciutto from a 90g pack, then stir through the meat mixture.

• STEP 3

Pour over 800g passata or half our basic tomato sauce recipe and 200ml hot beef stock. Add a little grated nutmeg, then season.

• STEP 4

Bring up to the boil, then simmer for 30 mins until the sauce looks rich.

• STEP 5

Heat the oven to 180C/160C fan/gas 4 and lightly oil an ovenproof dish (about 30 x 20cm).

• STEP 6

Spoon one third of the meat sauce into the dish, then cover with some fresh lasagne sheets from a 300g pack. Drizzle over roughly 130g ready-made or homemade white sauce.

• STEP 7

Repeat until you have three layers of pasta. Cover with the remaining 390g white sauce, making sure you can't see any pasta poking through.

• STEP 8

Scatter 125g torn mozzarella over the top.

• STEP 9

Arrange the rest of the prosciutto on top. Bake for 45 mins until the top is bubbling and lightly browned.

Haddock in tomato basil sauce

Ingredients

• 1 tbsp olive oil

• 1 onion, thinly sliced

• 1 small aubergine, about 250g/9oz, roughly chopped

• ½ tsp ground paprika

• 2 garlic cloves, crushed

• 400g can chopped tomato

• 1 tsp dark or light muscovado sugar

• 8 large basil leaves, plus a few extra for sprinkling

• 4 4x175g/6oz firm skinless white fish fillets, such as haddock

Directions

• STEP 1

Heat the olive oil in a large non-stick frying pan and stirfry the onion and aubergine. After about 4 minutes the vegetables will start to turn golden but won't be soft yet, so cover with a lid and let the vegetables steam-fry in their own juices for 6 minutes – this helps them to soften without needing to add any extra oil.

• STEP 2

Stir in the paprika, garlic, tomatoes and sugar with 1/2 tsp salt and cook for another 8-10 minutes, stirring, until onion and aubergine are tender.

• STEP 3

Scatter in the basil leaves then nestle the fish in the sauce, cover the pan and cook for 6-8 minutes until the fish flakes when tested with a knife and the flesh is firm but still moist. Tear over the rest of the basil and serve with a salad and crusty bread.

Antipasti salmon

Ingredients

• 100g sundried tomatoes in oil, drained and finely chopped

• small handful of basil, finely chopped, plus a few whole basil leaves

• small handful of dill, finely chopped, plus a few dill fronds to serve

• 2 tbsp capers, drained and rinsed

• 2 garlic cloves, crushed

• 1 lemon, zested and sliced

• 150g butter, softened

• 600g side of salmon, descaled and pin bones removed

• 3 tbsp pitted black olives

• 100g griddled artichoke hearts, drained and roughly chopped

Directions

• STEP 1

Put the tomatoes, half the herbs, 1 tbsp capers, the garlic, lemon zest and butter in a bowl and mash together with a spoon. Alternatively, tip into a food processor and blitz until combined. The flavoured butter will keep, chilled, for up to two days.

• STEP 2

Layer a sheet of baking parchment large enough to loosely wrap the salmon over an equally-sized sheet of foil. Place the salmon on top, then cut the fish into portions, without cutting all the way through to the skin, so the fillet remains intact.

Make the portions as big or small as you like, depending on how many you're feeding. Spread the flavoured butter over the salmon, then top with the remaining capers, the lemon slices, olives and artichokes. Wrap the foil and parchment over the salmon and scrunch the ends to seal, creating a loose parcel.

• STEP 3

To bake the salmon, heat the oven to 200C/180C fan/gas 6. Put the parcel on a baking tray and cook for 30 mins, then leave to stand for a few minutes before unwrapping. Alternatively, light the barbecue, wait for the flames to die down, put the parcel directly on the grill and cook for 8-15 mins, or until the salmon is cooked through. Check the salmon is cooked by pushing the flesh with a fork – it should easily flake. Serve on a platter, scattered with the remaining herbs and the buttery juices poured over.

Sticky onion & cheddar quiche

Ingredients

- 25g butter

- 500g small onion, (about 5 in total), halved and finely sliced

- 2 eggs

- 284ml pot double cream

- 140g mature cheddar, coarsely grated

For the pastry

- 280g plain flour, plus extra for dusting

• 140g cold butter

Directions

• STEP 1

To make the pastry, tip the flour and butter into a bowl, then rub together with your fingertips until completely mixed and crumbly. Add 8 tbsp cold water, then bring everything together with your hands until just combined. Roll into a ball and use straight away or chill for up to 2 days. The pastry can also be frozen for up to a month.

• STEP 2

Roll out the pastry on a lightly floured surface to a round about 5cm larger than a 25cm tin. Use your rolling pin to lift it up, then drape over the tart case so there is an overhang of pastry on the sides. Using a small ball of pastry scraps, push the pastry into the corners of the tin (see picture, above left). Chill in the fridge or freezer for 20 mins.

• STEP 3

Heat oven to 200C/fan 180C/gas 6. While the pastry is chilling, heat the butter in a pan and cook the onions for 20 mins, stirring occasionally, until they become sticky and golden. Remove from the heat.

• STEP 4

Lightly prick the base of the tart with a fork, line the tart case with a large circle of greaseproof paper or foil, then fill with baking beans. Blind-bake the tart for 20 mins, remove the paper and beans, then continue to cook for 5-10 mins until biscuit brown.

• STEP 5

Meanwhile, beat the eggs in a bowl, then gradually add the cream. Stir in the onions and half the cheese, then season with salt and pepper. Carefully tip the filling into the case, sprinkle with the rest of the cheese, then bake for 20-25 mins until set and golden. Leave to cool in the case, trim the edges of the pastry, then remove and serve in slices.

Steamed bass with pak choi

Ingredients

- small piece of ginger, peeled and sliced

- 2 garlic cloves, finely sliced

- 3 spring onions, finely sliced

- 2 tbsp soy sauce

- 1 tbsp sesame oil

- splash of sherry (optional)

- 2 x fillets sea bass

- 2 heads pak choi, quartered

Directions

- STEP 1

In a small bowl, mix all of the Ingredients, except the fish and the pak choi, together to make a soy mix. Line one tier of a two-tiered bamboo steamer loosely with foil. Lay the fish, skin side up, on the foil and spoon over the soy mix. Place the fish over simmering water and throw the pak choi into the second tier and cover it with a lid. Alternatively, add the pak choi to the fish layer after 2 mins of cooking – the closer the tier is to the steam, the hotter it is.

- STEP 2

Leave everything to steam for 6-8 mins until the pak choi has wilted and the fish is cooked. Divide the greens between two plates, then carefully lift out the fish. Lift the foil up and drizzle the tasty juices back over the fish.

Mackerel with orange & harissa glaze

Ingredients

- 2 x 300g/10oz mackerel, filleted and skin on or 4 x 75g/3oz mackerel fillets, skin on

- 2 tbsp plain flour

- ½ tsp smoked paprika

- 2 tbsp extra-virgin olive oil

- 1small orange, grated zest and juice

* 1-2 tsp harissa paste (to taste, as brands vary)

* 50g pine nut, toasted

* small bunch coriander, very roughly chopped

Directions

* STEP 1

Roll the mackerel fillets in the flour sifted with smoked paprika and seasoning. Shake off excess flour and set the fish aside in a single layer.

* STEP 2

Put 1 tbsp of the olive oil, the orange zest and juice and the harissa paste into a small bowl, and whisk together. Heat a frying pan with remaining olive oil until very hot. Fry the fish fillets for 5 mins, first on the skin side, then on the flesh side.

* STEP 3

When the fish is nearly cooked – it should look firm – pour over the orange and harissa glaze, bring to the boil and allow the liquid to bubble until sticky. Sprinkle over the pine nuts and coriander.

Strawberry & Tuna Spinach Salad

Ingredients

• 4 cups baby spinach

• ⅓ cup tuna salad

• ½ cup sliced white mushrooms

• ½ cup strawberries

• ¼ cup sliced red onion

• 2 tablespoons chopped celery

- 1 ½ tablespoons slivered almonds

- 1 tablespoon lemon juice

- ¼ cup mixed fresh fruit

- ¼ cup yogurt

Directions

1. Mix spinach, tuna salad, mushrooms, strawberries, and celery in a medium bowl. Drizzle lemon juice and sprinkle almonds on top.

2. Mix fruit and yogurt in a small bowl. Serve on the side.

Quinoa Chickpea Salad with Roasted Red Pepper Hummus Dressing

Ingredients

- 2 tablespoons hummus, original or roasted red pepper flavor

- 1 tablespoon lemon juice

- 1 tablespoon chopped roasted red pepper

- 2 cups mixed salad greens

- ½ cup cooked quinoa

- ½ cup chickpeas, rinsed

- 1 tablespoon unsalted sunflower seeds

- 1 tablespoon chopped fresh parsley

- Pinch of salt

- Pinch of ground pepper

Directions

1. Stir hummus, lemon juice and red peppers in a small dish. Thin with water to desired consistency for dressing.

2. Arrange greens, quinoa and chickpeas in a large bowl. Top with sunflower seeds, parsley, salt and pepper. Serve with the dressing.

BBQ Chicken Bowls

Ingredients

- 8 ounces Yukon Gold potatoes, cut into 1/2-in. pieces

- 1 tablespoon canola oil

- ⅞ teaspoon kosher salt, divided

- ½ teaspoon black pepper, divided

- 1 ½ tablespoons mayonnaise

- 1 tablespoon apple cider vinegar

- ½ teaspoon granulated sugar

- 2 cups angel hair coleslaw

- 2 (15 ounce) cans no-salt-added pinto beans, drained

- 2 cups shredded cooked chicken

- 6 tablespoons spicy barbecue sauce

- ½ cup water

- ½ cup fresh yellow corn kernels

- 1 tablespoon chopped fresh chives

Directions

1. Preheat oven to 450 degrees F. Toss potatoes with oil and 1/4 teaspoon each salt and pepper.

Spread on a rimmed baking sheet; roast until golden, about 15 minutes.

2. Whisk together mayonnaise, vinegar, sugar, 1/4 teaspoon salt, and 1/4 teaspoon pepper in a bowl. Add slaw, and toss to coat.

3. Combine beans, chicken, barbecue sauce, water, and 3/8 teaspoon salt in a saucepan; bring to a simmer over medium-high. Remove from heat; divide among 4 bowls. Top with potatoes, slaw, corn, and chives.

Green Goddess Salad with Chickpeas

Ingredients

Dressing

• 1 avocado, peeled and pitted

- 1 ½ cups buttermilk

- ¼ cup chopped fresh herbs, such as tarragon, sorrel, mint, parsley and/or cilantro

- 2 tablespoons rice vinegar

- ½ teaspoon salt

Salad

- 3 cups chopped romaine lettuce

- 1 cup sliced cucumber

- 1 (15 ounce) can chickpeas, rinsed

- ¼ cup diced low-fat Swiss cheese

- 6 cherry tomatoes, halved if desired

Directions

1. To prepare dressing: Place avocado, buttermilk, herbs, vinegar and salt in a blender. Puree until smooth.

2. To prepare salad: Toss lettuce and cucumber in a bowl with 1/4 cup of the dressing. Top with chickpeas, cheese and tomatoes. (Refrigerate the extra dressing for up to 3 days.)

Zucchini Noodle Bowls with Chicken Sausage & Pesto

Ingredients

• 2 teaspoons olive oil

• 6 ounces cooked Italian chicken sausage links (about 2), sliced into 1/2-inch pieces

• 1 pound zucchini noodles

- 1 (14 ounce) can no-salt-added cannellini beans, rinsed

- 1 (7 ounce) jar roasted red peppers, rinsed and sliced

- ½ cup refrigerated pesto

Directions

1. Heat oil in a nonstick skillet over medium heat. Add sausage and cook, stirring often, until browned and heated through, about 5 minutes.

2. Divide zucchini noodles among 4 single-serving containers with lids (about 2 cups per container). Top each with equal amounts of the sausage, beans, peppers and pesto.

3. To reheat, vent the lid and microwave on High until the sausage is steaming and the noodles are tender, 2 1/2 to 3 minutes.

Black Bean-Quinoa Bowl

Ingredients

- ¾ cup canned black beans, rinsed

- ⅔ cup cooked quinoa

- ¼ cup hummus

- 1 tablespoon lime juice

- ¼ medium avocado, diced

- 3 tablespoons pico de gallo

- 2 tablespoons chopped fresh cilantro

Directions

1. Combine beans and quinoa in a bowl. Stir hummus and lime juice together in a small bowl; thin with water to desired consistency. Drizzle the

hummus dressing over the beans and quinoa. Top with avocado, pico de gallo and cilantro.

DINNER RECIPES FOR PSC

Spinach & halloumi salad

Ingredients

- 250g halloumi cheese

- 200g bag spinach

- 2 large oranges

- 1 bunch mint, leaves only

Instructions

- STEP 1

Slice the halloumi and griddle for 3-4 mins each side until charred, then set aside. Tip the spinach and half the mint onto a large platter. Segment the oranges and pour any orange juice from the chopping board into a bowl, and squeeze the pith to get juices from there too. Scatter the orange pieces over the spinach. Chop the remaining mint and mix with the orange juice, 2 tbsp olive oil and some seasoning. Place the halloumi slices on top of the salad and pour the dressing over. Serve with warm flatbreads.

Healthier treacle sponge

Ingredients

- 2 tbsp rapeseed oil, plus ¼ tsp

- 5 tbsp golden syrup

- 1 small orange (½ tsp finely grated zest and 2 tbsp plus 1 tsp juice)

- 175g self-raising flour

- 1 ½ tsp baking powder

- 100g light muscovado sugar

- 25g ground almond

- 2 large eggs

- 175g natural yogurt

- 1 tsp black treacle

- 25g butter, melted

Instructions

- STEP 1

Heat oven to 180C/160C fan/gas 4. Brush 6 x 200ml pudding tins with the ¼ tsp oil, then sit them on a baking tray. Stir together 4 tbsp of the golden syrup, the orange zest and 2 tbsp orange juice and spoon a little into the bottom of each tin (step 1).

• STEP 2

Tip the flour, baking powder, sugar (breaking up any lumps with your fingers) and ground almonds into a large mixing bowl and make a dip in the centre. Beat the eggs in a separate bowl, then stir in the yogurt and treacle. Pour this mixture, along with the melted butter and remaining 2 tbsp oil, into the dry mixture (step 2) and stir together briefly with a large metal spoon, just so everything is well combined. Divide the mixture evenly between the tins (step 3). Bake for 20-25 mins or until the puddings have risen to the top of the tins and feel firm.

• STEP 3

Mix together the remaining 1 tbsp golden syrup and 1 tsp orange juice to drizzle over as a sauce. To serve, if the pudding tops have peaked slightly, slice off to level so they sit upright when turned out. Loosen around the sides with a round-bladed knife (step 4), then turn them out onto plates. Scrape out any syrupy bits remaining in the tins and put on top of the puddings, then drizzle a little of the syrup sauce over and around each one.

Gnocchi traybake with lemony ricotta

Ingredients

- 500g gnocchi

- 1 courgette, halved, then sliced into chunky pieces

- 100g baby plum tomatoes, halved

- 100g artichokes in oil, plus 2 tbsp of the oil

- 2 garlic cloves, unpeeled, lightly bashed

- ½ tsp chilli flakes

- 85g ricotta

- 1 lemon, zested, then sliced into wedges

- 10g basil, roughly chopped

Instructions

- STEP 1

Heat the oven to 220C/200C fan/gas 8. Tip the gnocchi, courgette and tomatoes into a large roasting tray. Add the artichokes and oil, the bashed garlic cloves and chilli flakes, and season well with salt and freshly ground black pepper. Mix all the Ingredients together with your hands, then bake for 30-35 mins until the gnocchi are crisp at the edges and the veg is soft.

• STEP 2

Meanwhile, mix the ricotta and lemon zest together in a small bowl, then season with salt and pepper to taste. Dot this over the gnocchi and sprinkle over the basil.

• STEP 3

Divide the gnocchi between two bowls, mixing them well so the ricotta breaks down to make a creamy sauce. Serve with the lemon wedges for squeezing over.

Root vegetable tatin with candied nuts & blue cheese

Ingredients

• 500g block puff pastry

• 3 slim carrots, about 12-13 cm long, halved lengthways

• 3 slim parsnips about 12-13 cm long, halved lengthways plus 1 large parsnip, peeled and grated

• 2 tbsp olive oil

• 2 heaped tbsp slightly salted butter

• 5 banana shallots, 3 halved lengthways, 2 thinly sliced

• small bunch sage, leaves picked and finely chopped

• 4 rosemary sprigs, leaves picked and finely chopped

• 2 garlic cloves, finely grated or crushed

- 100g caster sugar

- 125ml red wine vinegar

- 100g blue cheese, crumbled (we used Cropwell Bishop)

For the candied nuts

- 50g walnuts, roughly chopped

- 25g caster sugar

- 2 tsp butter

- 3 rosemary sprigs

Instructions

- STEP 1

Heat oven to 200C/180C fan/gas 6. Roll out the pastry to just larger than a 30cm diameter ovenproof frying pan and use the pan as a template to cut out a round of pastry. Leave in the fridge, or a cool place while you prepare everything else.

• STEP 2

Bring a pan of water to the boil, add the carrots and parsnips and cook for 5 mins. Drain and set aside to dry off slightly. Heat the oil and 1 tbsp of the butter in your pan and cook the sliced shallots and grated parsnips for 1-2 mins over a medium-high heat until just starting to brown, then add a good splash of water to the pan, stir to scrape up any brown bits, turn the heat down slightly, cover and cook for 4-5 mins, stirring every so often. The parsnips should be tender. Add the herbs and garlic and cook for another minute, then tip into a bowl, scraping out as well as you can. Season a little and set aside.

- STEP 3

Add the sugar and vinegar to the pan and bring to the boil. Cook for a few minutes until syrupy, then stir in the remaining butter. Set aside to cool slightly, then arrange the vegetables in the pan, fanning them out. Top with the herby shallot and parsnip mixture, pushing it into any spaces there may be. Lay the pastry over the top of the vegetables and push in the edges a little. Place in the oven and bake for 30-35 mins until puffed and deep golden brown.

- STEP 4

While the tart bakes, put the nuts, sugar and butter in a small frying pan with a pinch of salt. Cook over a medium-high heat for about 5 mins, stirring, until the sugar has dissolved and coated the nuts. Add the rosemary for the last minute. Tip out onto a piece of baking parchment and leave to cool for a few minutes.

• STEP 5

Once the tart is baked, remove from the oven and carefully turn out onto a serving board. Scrape out any bits that are left in the tin and add back to the tart. Bash the nuts to break them up and scatter over, along with the crumbled cheese.

Vegan beetroot bourguignon

Ingredients

• 100g green lentils

• 6-8 small beetroot (450g unprepped), peeled and halved if small, or quartered if larger

• 1 tbsp vegetable oil

- 1 onion, cut into wedges

- 3 carrots, peeled and cut into large chunks on an angle

- 1 tsp dried thyme

- 2 tbsp tomato purée

- 1 tbsp balsamic or red wine vinegar

- 1 tsp yeast extract (optional)

- 1 tbsp soy sauce

- 300ml vegan red wine

- 300ml vegetable stock

- 250g chestnut mushrooms, quartered

- 2 bay leaves

- crusty bread, to serve (optional)

Instructions

• STEP 1

Soak the lentils in a bowl of cold water for 40 mins. Meanwhile, heat the oven to 230C/210C fan/gas 8. Put the beetroot in a large, deep flameproof casserole dish with the oil, onion, carrots and thyme. Mix together and season.

• STEP 2

Roast for 35 mins, mixing all the vegetables halfway through until starting to go crisp (they don't need to be cooked all the way through at this point). Remove the dish from the oven and put on the hob over a medium heat. Turn the oven down to 200C/180C fan/gas 6.

• STEP 3

Drain the lentils and add to the dish. Mix in the rest of the Ingredients, and a good crack of black pepper. Bring to the boil, then take off the heat and cover with a lid.

• STEP 4

Transfer to the oven and cook for 55 mins-1 hr until the lentils are cooked, the veg is soft with a little bite and the liquid has thickened and reduced. Serve in bowls with bread for dunking, if you like.

Delicious Summer egg salad with basil & peas

Ingredients

• 150g new potatoes, thickly sliced

• 160g French beans, trimmed

- 160g frozen peas

- 3 eggs

- 160g romaine lettuce, roughly torn into pieces

For the dressing

- 1 tbsp extra virgin olive oil

- 2 tsp cider vinegar

- ½ tsp English mustard powder

- 2 tbsp chopped mint

- 3 tbsp chopped basil

- 1 garlic clove, finely grated

- 1 tbsp capers

Instructions

- STEP 1

Cook the potatoes in a pan of simmering water for 5 mins. Add the beans and cook 5 mins more, then tip in the peas and cook for 2 mins until all the vegetables are just tender. Meanwhile, boil the eggs in another pan for 8 mins. Drain and run under cold water, then carefully shell and halve.

- STEP 2

Mix all the dressing Ingredients together in a large bowl with a good grinding of black pepper, crushing the herbs and capers with the back of a spoon to intensify their flavours.

- STEP 3

Mix the warm vegetables into the dressing to coat, then add the lettuce and toss everything together.

Pile onto plates, top with the eggs and grind over some black pepper to serve.

Spicy chickpea stew

Ingredients

- 1 tbsp rapeseed oil

- 2 onions (320g), roughly chopped

- 2 green peppers, deseeded and cut into cubes

- 2 tsp hot chilli powder

- 1 tbsp ground coriander

- 1 tsp ground cumin

- 500ml carton passata

- 2 x 400g cans chickpeas

* 2 tsp vegetable bouillon powder

* 40g flame raisins

* ½ lemon, juiced, flesh scooped out and white pith removed, then zest finely chopped (you'll need 2 tsp)

* 350g cauliflower florets

* 15g parsley, chopped

* 140g wholemeal couscous

* 40g toasted flaked almonds

Instructions

* STEP 1

Heat the oil in a large lidded pan over a medium heat and fry the onions for 10 mins, stirring often until golden. Stir in the peppers and cook for 5 mins more.

• STEP 2

Add the chilli powder, coriander and cumin, stir briefly, then tip in the passata and chickpeas along with the liquid from the cans.

• STEP 3

Stir in the bouillon powder, raisins and lemon zest, then add the cauliflower. Cover tightly and simmer over a medium heat for 15-20 mins until the cauliflower is tender. Stir in half the parsley.

• STEP 4

Meanwhile, put the couscous in a heatproof bowl and pour over 175ml boiling water from the kettle. Stir in the lemon juice, then cover and let stand for about 10 mins until the couscous has absorbed the liquid and is tender. Stir in the toasted flaked almonds and most of the remaining parsley.

• STEP 5

Divide half the couscous between two plates and top with half the chickpea stew and the rest of the parsley. Leave the remainder to cool for another day. Will keep covered and chilled for up to three days. Reheat the stew in a pan over a low heat with a splash of water until piping hot. Reheat the couscous in the microwave.

Mustard salmon & veg bake with horseradish sauce

Ingredients

• 4 parsnips, sliced lengthways

• 4 small raw beetroot, thickly sliced

- 6 carrots, sliced lengthways

- 2 tbsp olive oil

- 4 x 125g/4½oz pieces salmon with skin

- 2 tbsp grainy mustard

- 2 tbsp hot horseradish

- 150ml crème fraîche

- 1 tbsp cider vinegar

- 1 tbsp chopped dill

Directions

- STEP 1

Heat oven to 200C/180C fan/gas 6. Toss all the vegetables with the oil and season well. Spread in a single layer on 2 baking trays (or 1 very large tray) and roast for 30 mins.

- STEP 2

Season the salmon and spread over the mustard. In the final 10 mins of cooking the veg, add the salmon to the trays.

- STEP 3

In a small bowl, mix together the horseradish, crème fraîche, vinegar, dill and some seasoning. Serve the salmon with the sauce and veg.

Hake fish cakes with mustard middles

Ingredients

For the fish cakes

- 450g floury potatoes, cut into chunks (we used Rooster potatoes)

- 1 bay leaf

- a few peppercorns

- 450g skinless hake fillet, cut into 4

- bunch spring onions, finely shredded

- 1 whole nutmeg

- 3 tbsp plain flour, seasoned

- 1 egg

- 100g fresh breadcrumbs

- 2l vegetable oil, for deep-frying

- salad leaves, to serve

- lemon wedges, to serve

For the mustard middles

- 100g full-fat crème fraîche

- 50g strong cheddar, grated

- 1 egg yolk (reserve the white)

- 1 tbsp wholegrain mustard

Directions

- STEP 1

Mix all the mustard middle Ingredients together. Drape cling film across a muffin tin, then spoon the mix into 4 of the wells. Freeze for 30 mins or until solid.

- STEP 2

Put the potatoes, bay leaf and peppercorns in a pan of cold water, bring to the boil and cook for 20 mins or until tender. Remove and allow to steam-dry in a colander. Add the fish to the water and simmer for 5 mins until it is just cooked through at the thickest part.

• STEP 3

Mash the potatoes and stir in the spring onions, a little freshly grated nutmeg and some seasoning. Drain the hake, then flake it into the mash. Gently mix everything together and leave to cool.

• STEP 4

Divide the fish mixture into 4. Shape 1 fish cake at a time, moulding it into a ball. Make a well in the centre of the ball and push a frozen mustard middle into it, then shape the mash around it to make a smooth hockey-puck shape. Repeat with the remaining fish, then freeze for 15 mins.

• STEP 5

Using 3 shallow bowls, add the flour to one; put the egg and reserved egg white in another, and the breadcrumbs in the third. Beat the eggs with some seasoning. Thoroughly coat the fishcakes first in the flour, then the egg , then the breadcrumbs. Freeze the fish cakes until firm. Can be frozen for up to 1 month – defrost in the fridge for 2 hrs before cooking.

• STEP 6

When ready to cook, heat the oil to 180C in a large, deep saucepan (or use a fat fryer) and the oven to 190C/170C fan/gas 5. Fry the fish cakes for 7 mins, turning halfway, until crisp. Drain on kitchen paper, transfer to a baking sheet and bake for 5 mins (15 mins from frozen) so the middles are hot. Serve with dressed leaves and a lemon wedge.

Baked sea bream with tomatoes & coriander

Ingredients

- 4 large potatoes, about 1kg/2lb 4oz

- 2 garlic cloves, finely chopped

- pinch dried chilli flakes

- pinch saffron

- 1 bunch coriander, roughly chopped

- 4 whole sea bream, cleaned and gutted

- 1 tbsp olive oil, plus extra for greasing

- juice 2 limes

- 125ml white wine

- handful sundried tomatoes

- handful pine nuts, toasted

- 4 thin slices pancetta or smoked streaky bacon

Directions

- STEP 1

Heat the oven to 200C/180C fan/gas 6. Slice the potatoes thinly, put in a large saucepan and cover with cold salted water. Bring to the boil and drain, then lay onto the base of a lightly oiled large baking tray. Scatter over the garlic, chilli, saffron and a little of the coriander.

- STEP 2

Slash the fish through the flesh down to the bone – this allows it to cook evenly and quicker than normal. Season and rub with the olive oil. Lay the fish on the potatoes and top with the lime juice, wine, tomatoes and pine nuts. Lay the pancetta slices over the fish and bake for 20-25 mins or until the fish is cooked through. Check by pulling out one of the fins on the back, it should come away easily. Serve the fish scattered with the remaining coriander.

Herby fish fingers

Ingredients

- 50g crustless stale white bread

- finely grated zest of a large lemon

- 2 tbsp each roughly chopped fresh dill, fresh chives and fresh parsley

- 500g skinless lemon sole fillets

- 2 tbsp seasoned flour

- 1 egg, beaten

* vegetable oil, for shallow frying

Directions

* STEP 1

Pulse the bread to coarse crumbs in the food processor. Add the lemon zest, herbs and a pinch of salt, and pulse to make bright green, fine breadcrumbs.

* STEP 2

Cut the lemon sole into thick strips, about 3 x 10cm. Dust each fish piece with the fl our, shake off any excess, then dip into the egg then the breadcrumbs. At this stage, they can be cooked straight away, kept in the fridge for a few hours, or frozen.

* STEP 3

To serve, heat about 1cm of oil in a large frying pan. Once it's nice and hot, fry the fish fingers a few at a time for 1-2 mins on each side. Drain on kitchen paper, and keep warm while you continue with the rest. When they are all cooked, serve straight away with the oven-roasted chips and tartare sauce.

Salmon & lemon mini fish cakes

Ingredients

- 2 large baking potatoes

- 2 tbsp olive oil

- grated zest and juice ½ lemon

- 1 egg yolk

- 140g smoked salmon trimmings, plus extra to serve

- 1 tbsp chopped parsley, plust extra

- 2 tbsp gluten-free flour mixed with 1 tsp coarsely ground pepper

- a little oil, for frying

Directions

- STEP 1

Microwave potatoes on high for 10 mins until tender. Leave to cool for 5 mins, scoop the flesh in a bowl, then mash and leave to cool. Season with olive oil, lemon zest and juice to taste, then mix in the egg, salmon and parsley. Shape into small rounds 3cm wide and 1cm deep. Chill for 15 mins.

- STEP 2

Dust each cake with the peppered flour, then fry over a low heat in a little oil for 2-3 mins on each side. Drain on kitchen paper and serve garnished with salmon and parsley.

Spinach, Mushroom & Egg Casserole

Ingredients

• 2 tablespoons extra-virgin olive oil

• 1 pound cremini mushrooms, trimmed and sliced

• 5 medium cloves garlic, finely chopped

• 2 teaspoons dry mustard

• 1 teaspoon onion powder

• 1 teaspoon salt

- 5 ounces baby spinach

- 12 large eggs

- ¾ cup half-and-half

- 1 ½ cups shredded Gruyère cheese, preferably cave-aged (see Tip), divided

- 2 teaspoons fresh thyme leaves

Directions

1. Preheat oven to 375°F. Coat a 9-by-13-inch baking dish with cooking spray. Heat oil in a large skillet over medium-high heat. Add mushrooms in an even layer; cook, undisturbed, until starting to brown, 5 to 6 minutes. Stir and continue to cook, undisturbed, until golden brown on the bottom, about 3 minutes. Stir and continue to cook, stirring occasionally, until the mushrooms are browned all over and the liquid has evaporated, about 3

minutes. Add garlic, dry mustard, onion powder and salt; cook, stirring constantly, until fragrant, about 1 minute. Add spinach and cook, stirring constantly, until the spinach wilts, 1 to 2 minutes. Set aside to cool slightly, about 10 minutes.

2. Crack eggs into a large bowl and whisk until completely smooth. Add half-and-half and whisk until combined. Reserve 1/2 cup of the vegetable mixture; scatter the remaining mixture in the prepared baking dish. Sprinkle evenly with 3/4 cup Gruyère. Pour the egg mixture over the top. Sprinkle evenly with the remaining 3/4 cup Gruyère and the reserved 1/2 cup vegetable mixture. Bake until puffed, golden brown and just set, 30 to 35 minutes. Let cool slightly, about 10 minutes. Sprinkle with thyme before serving.

Tip

Cave-aged Gruyère is aged for at least a year in caves that provide the perfect environment for aging which intensifies the flavor and hardens the texture of the cheese. Look for it in well-stocked supermarkets, specialty cheese shops or online. While cave-aged Gruyère adds depth of flavor to this recipe, regular Gruyère will work well too.

Loaded Cucumber & Avocado Sandwich

Ingredients

• 3 tablespoons shredded extra-sharp Cheddar cheese

• 2 tablespoons ricotta cheese

• 4 teaspoons finely sliced chives

• 2 teaspoons lemon juice

• Ground pepper to taste

• 2 slices whole-wheat sandwich bread, lightly toasted

• ⅓ cup thinly sliced cucumber

• ¼ cup thinly sliced red bell pepper

• ⅓ avocado, sliced

Directions

1. Stir Cheddar, ricotta, chives, lemon juice, salt and pepper together in a small bowl. Spread half the mixture on each slice of toast. Layer one slice with cucumber, pepper and avocado, then top with the other slice, spread-side down.

Gochujang-Glazed Salmon with Garlic Spinach

Ingredients

- 2 tablespoons gochujang

- 1 tablespoon mirin

- 2 tablespoons reduced-sodium tamari, divided

- 1 tablespoon honey

- 1 ½ teaspoons toasted sesame oil, divided

- 4 cloves garlic, grated, divided

- 2 teaspoons grated fresh ginger

- 1 ¼ pounds salmon, preferably wild-caught, cut into 4 portions

- 8 cups baby spinach

- Sesame seeds & sliced scallions for garnish

Directions

1. Position a rack in upper third of oven; preheat broiler to high. Line a baking sheet with foil and coat with cooking spray.

2. Whisk gochujang, mirin, 1 tablespoon tamari, honey, 1/2 teaspoon sesame oil, 1/4 of the garlic and ginger in a small bowl. Pat salmon dry and place skin-side down on the prepared pan. Brush the salmon with the glaze. Broil until the salmon is just cooked through, 5 to 8 minutes, depending on thickness.

3. Meanwhile, heat the remaining 1 teaspoon sesame oil in a large skillet over medium-low heat. Add the remaining 3 cloves garlic and cook, stirring, until fragrant and just starting to brown, about 3 minutes. Add spinach and cook, stirring,

until wilted and the pan is dry, about 3 minutes. Remove from heat and stir in the remaining 1 tablespoon tamari.

4. Serve the salmon over the spinach.

SIDE DISH RECIPES FOR PSC

Cheesy roasted courgettes

Ingredients

- 4 courgettes, halved lengthways

- 250g tub ricotta

- zest 1 lemon

- 1 chilli, deseeded and finely chopped

- handful chopped herbs, such as mint, parsley and basil

- 4 tbsp dried breadcrumbs

Directions

- STEP 1

Heat oven to 200C/180C fan/gas 6. Use a teaspoon to scoop the seeds from the middle of each courgette half, then place them in a large baking tray.

• STEP 2

Mix together the ricotta, zest, chilli and herbs, and season with salt and pepper. Pile the stuffing into the courgettes and top with breadcrumbs. Bake for 35 mins until the courgettes are tender and the topping is golden and crisp.

Baked feta with sesame & honey

Ingredients

• 1 tbsp sesame seeds, toasted

• 200g block feta

• 2 tbsp honey, plus extra to serve

• 1 tsp roughly chopped oregano

• olive oil, for drizzling

• warmed pitta breads, to serve

Directions

• STEP 1

Heat the oven to 200C/180C fan/gas 6, or if using an air-fryer, heat to 180C for 3 mins. Put the sesame seeds in a shallow dish and brush the block of feta all over with the honey. Carefully press the honey-coated feta into the sesame seeds, turning so that it's well crusted with seeds.

• STEP 2

Put the feta in a baking dish (it should fit snugly), then sprinkle over the oregano and a pinch of sea salt. Drizzle with some olive oil. Bake in the oven for 15-20 mins, or cook in the air-fryer for 15 mins until the feta is soft, then drizzle with a little extra honey and serve with the pitta breads on the side.

Smoked haddock & cheddar fishcakes with watercress sauce

Ingredients

- 425g floury potatoes, cut into large chunks

- 1 bay leaf

- 6 peppercorns

- small bunch flat-leaf parsley, leaves and stalks separated

- 225g smoked haddock fillets, skin on (we used dyed haddock to give the mash a lovely golden colour)

- 200g unsmoked haddock fillets, skin on

- 75g mature British cheddar, grated

- 4 spring onions, 0.5 very finely sliced, 0.5 roughly chopped

- 50g plain flour

- 2 medium eggs, beaten

- 100g fresh breadcrumbs

- sunflower oil, for frying

- 50g watercress (weighed after discarding the thickest stalks)

- 4 tbsp rapeseed oil

• 2 lemons, 1 juiced, 1 cut into small wedges to serve (optional)

Directions

• STEP 1

Put the potatoes, bay leaf, peppercorns and parsley stalks in a big pan of cold water. Cover with a lid, bring to the boil and cook for 15 mins until tender. Using a slotted spoon, transfer the potatoes to a colander and leave to steam-dry. Turn the heat down, add the fish and poach gently for 5 mins until it flakes easily. Tip the potatoes into a big bowl and put the fish in the colander to drain for a few mins.

• STEP 2

Add the cheese, some pepper and a little salt to the potatoes and mash well. Flake in about half the fish, discarding the skin and bones, and mash in too. Flake in the remaining fish in big chunks, scatter over the sliced spring onions and gently mix together. Roll the mixture into golf-ball-sized cakes.

• STEP 3

Tip the flour onto a plate and season. Tip the egg and breadcrumbs into 2 shallow bowls each. Roll each fishcake first in the flour, then the egg, then the breadcrumbs. Sit on some parchment-lined trays that fit in your fridge. Chill for at least 1 hr or up to 24 hrs.

• STEP 4

Fill a deep frying pan with 1-2cm of sunflower oil, heat until shimmering, then brown a few fishcakes at a time, turning regularly. If the oil gets too crumby, change halfway through. You can serve them straight away, or cool and chill for up to 24 hrs in the fridge, then simply warm for 30 mins in an oven at 180C/160C fan/ gas 4 before the party.

• STEP 5

Make the dipping sauce up to 1 hr before serving – put the roughly chopped spring onions, the parsley leaves, watercress, rapeseed oil, 2 tbsp lemon juice and 5 tbsp water in a food processor or blender. Whizz to the consistency of single cream.

• STEP 6

Pile the warm fishcakes onto a platter with a bowl of watercress sauce on the side and some lemon wedges for squeezing over, if you like.

Lemon & coriander couscous

Ingredients

- 250g couscous

- grated zest of a lemon

- 2 x 20g packs fresh coriander

- 4 tbsp raisins

- 4 tbsp toasted pine nuts

Directions

- STEP 1

Prepare 250g couscous with boiling water or stock, according to the packet's instructions.

- STEP 2

Add the lemon zest, fresh coriander, raisins and pine nuts. Season well and drizzle with plenty of olive oil. Goes really well with fish or lamb.

Perfect roast potatoes

Ingredients

- 16 potatoes the best ones to use are Desirée, as they hold their shape, but King Edward and Maris Piper are also good

- 2 tbsp plain flour

- 140g goose fat or duck fat or dripping

- 3 tbsp sunflower oil or vegetable oil

Directions

- STEP 1

Heat oven to 190C/fan 170C/gas 5. Peel the potatoes and cut in half; if very large, cut into quarters, or leave whole if they are small. Tip into a saucepan, cover with cold water, then bring to the boil. Set the timer and boil for exactly 2 mins. Drain the potatoes well, then toss in the colander to fluff up their surfaces, sprinkling over the flour as you go.

• STEP 2

Place a large, sturdy roasting tray over a fairly high heat, then tip in the fat and oil. When sizzling, lower in the potatoes carefully, then gently brown in the hot fat for about 5 mins so all the sides are covered with oil.

• STEP 3

Roast undisturbed for 20 mins, then remove from the oven and gently turn them over with a fish slice. Place the tray on the hob to heat the oil, then return to the oven and cook for another 20 mins. Turn again, putting the tray back on the hob to heat the oil. Give them a final 20 mins in the oven, by which time you should have perfect roast potatoes.

Courgette & anchovy salad

Ingredients

- ¼ tsp fennel seed

- juice and zest ½ lemon

- 1 tbsp extra-virgin olive oil, plus extra for drizzling

- 1 garlic clove, crushed

- 1 large courgette, thinly sliced on the diagonal

- 50g rocket

- 2 anchovy fillets, halved

Directions

• STEP 1

Toast the fennel seeds in a small frying pan over a low-medium heat for 1 min, or until they release their aroma. Bash them lightly using a pestle and mortar. Mix the lemon juice, fennel seeds, oil and garlic in a large bowl, then stir in the courgette. Season and set aside to marinate for 30 mins.

• STEP 2

Toss through the rocket and transfer to a platter. Top with the anchovy fillets. Scatter with lemon zest and serve with an extra drizzle of olive oil.

Barbecued fennel with black olive dressing

Ingredients

• 2 fennel bulbs, sliced lengthways into 1cm-thick pieces

• 1 ½ tbsp olive oil

• 2 tbsp finely chopped black Kalamata olive

• 1 garlic clove, crushed

• juice 1 lemon

• small handful each parsley and basil, finely chopped

Directions

• STEP 1

Heat a BBQ or griddle pan. Toss the fennel in 1 tbsp of the oil, coating well. Cook for 5 mins on each side until golden brown and charred.

• STEP 2

To make the dressing, put the olives, garlic, lemon juice and remaining oil in a bowl. Add the chopped herbs and combine. Lay the fennel on a platter and pour over the dressing. Eat warm or at room temperature.

Apricot pancakes with honey butter

Ingredients

For the butter

• 100g butter, softened

• 2 tbsp clear honey

For the pancakes

• 140g self-raising flour

• pinch bicarbonate of soda

- 25g caster sugar

- 1 egg

- 150ml milk

- handful ready-to-eat dried apricots, finely chopped

- oil, for frying

Directions

- STEP 1

For the honey butter, beat the butter with the honey and spoon onto a large piece of cling film. Squeeze into a sausage shape, then wrap tightly and chill until ready to use. Will keep in the fridge for up to a month.

- STEP 2

Sift the flour, bicarbonate of soda and a small pinch of salt into a bowl, then stir through the sugar and make a well in the centre. Beat together the egg and milk, then gradually pour into the well, stirring slowly, to avoid creating lumps. Stir in the apricots.

• STEP 3

Heat a non-stick frying pan over a low heat and add a little oil. Drop in 4 tablespoonfuls of batter and cook for 1 min or until the surface of each pancake is covered in bubbles. Flip with a palette knife or fish slice, then cook for a further min. Repeat with the remaining batter. Serve warm or leave to cool, then toast and spread with the honey butter to serve

Harissa cauliflower pilaf

Ingredients

- 300g basmati rice

- 1 red onion, finely sliced

- 2 lemons, 1 juiced, 1 cut into wedges

- 2 tsp sugar

- 4 tbsp harissa

- 1 garlic clove, crushed

- 1 tbsp olive oil

- 1 large or 2 medium cauliflower, broken into large florets, stalk chopped, large leaves roughly chopped

- pinch of saffron

- 2 bay leaves

- 700ml hot vegan vegetable stock

- 100g sultanas

- 100g flaked almonds, toasted until golden brown

- ½ small bunch of dill, chopped, plus extra to serve

- 400g can chickpeas, drained and rinsed

- 50g pomegranate seeds (optional)

Directions

- STEP 1

Wash the rice really well, then leave to soak in cold water for 1 hr. Put the onion in a small bowl and toss with the lemon juice, the sugar and a pinch of salt. Leave to pickle while you make the pilaf.

• STEP 2

Heat the oven to 200C/180C fan/gas 6. Whisk 2 tbsp harissa, the garlic and oil in a large bowl, then add the cauliflower and toss to coat in the sauce. Season, then tip into a roasting tin and roast for 30 mins until tender and golden.

• STEP 3

Meanwhile, mix the saffron, bay leaves, stock and 2 tbsp harissa in a pan over a very low heat to keep warm while the cauli roasts.

• STEP 4

Remove the cauli from the oven, tip into a dish and squeeze over the juice from one of the lemon wedges. Drain the rice and tip into the roasting tin. Pour over the infused stock, and mix well. Stir in the sultanas, half the almonds, the dill, chickpeas, and half the cauliflower. Cover the tin with a double layer of foil, sealing well, then bake for 30 mins until the rice is tender and stock is absorbed.

• STEP 5

Fluff up the rice with a fork, then fold in the remaining cauliflower (this creates a contrast of cauli textures). Scatter over the extra dill, the remaining almonds, the pomegranate seeds, if using, the pickled red onions and remaining lemon wedges to squeeze over.

Quinoa, pea & avocado salad

Ingredients

• 100g frozen peas

• juice 1 lemon

* 2 tbsp olive oil

* ½ small pack mint, leaves only, chopped

* ½ small pack chives, snipped

* 250g pack ready-to-eat red & white quinoa mix
(we used Merchant Gourmet)

* 1 avocado, stoned, peeled and chopped into
chunks

* 75g bag pea shoots

Directions

* STEP 1

Put the peas in a large heatproof bowl, pour over
just-boiled water, then set aside.

* STEP 2

Pour the lemon juice into a small bowl and whisk in some seasoning. Keep whisking as you slowly add the olive oil, followed by the mint and chives.

• STEP 3

Drain the peas and tip into a large serving dish. Stir in the quinoa, breaking up any clumps. Pour over the dressing, then fold in the avocado and pea shoots. Serve immediately.

Spicy salmon tabbouleh

Ingredients

• 400g bulgur wheat

• 500g salmon fillet, pin-boned

• 3 tbsp sunflower oil

• 2 onions, finely chopped

- 5cm piece ginger, peeled and finely chopped

- 2 tbsp curry paste (we used korma)

- 300g Greek yogurt

- juice 1 lemon, plus 2 cut into wedges, to serve

- 300g smoked salmon

- handful coriander or parsley, roughly chopped

Directions

- STEP 1

Cook the bulgur wheat in plenty of salted water for 7 mins (or follow pack instructions). Drain, tip into a large bowl and leave to cool. Put the salmon fillet on a foil-lined grill, brush lightly with oil and season. Grill for 7-10 mins, turning halfway, until the fish flakes easily. Cool.

• STEP 2

Heat the remaining oil, add the onions and ginger, and fry for about 5 mins until softened and lightly coloured. Stir in the curry paste and cook for 1 min, stirring. Remove from the heat and stir in the yogurt, lemon juice and some seasoning. Leave to cool.

• STEP 3

Skin and flake the salmon fillet. Cut the smoked salmon into strips. Add the fresh salmon and half the smoked salmon to the bulgur wheat with the dressing and half the coriander. Stir everything together lightly, so as not to break up the salmon flakes too much. Tip onto a serving platter and scatter over the remaining smoked salmon strips and coriander. Add the lemon wedges and serve.

Warm mackerel & beetroot salad

Ingredients

- 450g new potato, cut into bite-size pieces

- 3 smoked mackerel fillets, skinned

- 250g pack cooked beetroot

- 100g bag mixed salad leaves

- 2 celery sticks, finely sliced

- 50g walnut pieces

For the dressing

- 6 tbsp good-quality salad dressing

- 2 tsp creamed horseradish sauce

Directions

• STEP 1

Boil the potatoes for 12-15 mins until just tender. Meanwhile, flake the mackerel fillets into large pieces and cut the beetroot into bite-size chunks.

• STEP 2

Drain the potatoes and cool slightly. Mix the salad dressing and horseradish sauce together in a salad bowl and season. Tip in the potatoes – they should still be warm.

• STEP 3

Add the salad leaves, mackerel, beetroot, celery and walnuts, and toss gently. Serve with crusty bread.

Courgettes with mint & ricotta

Ingredients

- 2 tbsp olive oil

- 2 tsp unsalted butter

- 4 large courgettes (we used a mixture of green and yellow), sliced

- zest and juice 1 lemon

- pinch of chilli flakes

- 70g ricotta

- extra virgin olive oil, for drizzling

- handful mint leaves, picked and roughly chopped

Directions

• STEP 1

Heat a large, heavy non-stick frying pan or cast-iron skillet over a medium heat. Heat 1 tbsp of the oil and 1 tsp butter together and add half the courgettes in one layer. Cook for 2 mins, then turn the heat down to medium-low and cook for 5 more mins untouched, until the underside has a nice colour. Flip the courgettes, then grate over some lemon zest, pour over half the lemon juice and season with salt, pepper and chilli flakes. Cook for a further 5 mins or until very tender. Repeat the process with the remaining slices of courgette.

• STEP 2

Transfer to a platter and top with spoonfuls of ricotta. Drizzle over some extra virgin olive oil and scatter over the mint to serve.

Stir-fried greens with fish sauce

Ingredients

- ½ head Savoy cabbage

- 125g purple sprouting or Tenderstem broccoli

- 2 tbsp groundnut oil

- 4-6 garlic cloves, finely sliced

- 75g baby spinach

- 2 tbsp fish sauce, plus extra for seasoning

- 1 tsp caster sugar

Directions

- STEP 1

Remove any discoloured or coarse leaves from the cabbage, then halve it. Remove the hard central ribs and discard them, then shred the leaves. If using purple sprouting broccoli, halve any thicker stems lengthways.

• STEP 2

Heat the oil in a wok. Stir-fry the broccoli for 1 min, then add the garlic and cabbage and cook until the garlic is a pale gold colour. Quickly add the spinach and fish sauce and turn the veg over – the moisture should come out of the spinach and boil off quickly. Add the sugar and toss the vegetables again, then add a little more fish sauce, if you like.

Fish o'leekie

Ingredients

- 1 leek, finely sliced

- 500ml vegetable stock

- 300g basmati rice

- 500g cod or haddock fillet, skinned and cut into large chunks

- handful parsley, roughly chopped

- finely grated zest and juice 1 lemon

Directions

- STEP 1

Put the leek in a large microwave dish with 4 tbsp of the stock. Cover the dish with cling film, pierce the film with a knife, then microwave on High for 5 mins.

- STEP 2

Uncover the dish, then stir the rice and remaining stock into the leek. Re-cover with cling film, pierce and microwave on High for another 10 mins, stirring halfway through until the rice is very nearly cooked.

• STEP 3

Gently stir in the fish chunks, cover the dish with cling film again, then pierce and cook for a further 5 mins until the fish flakes easily and the rice is tender. Stir in the parsley, lemon zest and juice. Leave to stand for 2 mins before serving.

Chapter 5: Living with PSC

Lifestyle and home remedies

If you've been diagnosed with primary sclerosing cholangitis, take steps to care for your liver, such as:

Don't drink alcohol.

Get vaccinated against hepatitis A and B.

Use care with chemicals at home and at work.

Maintain a healthy weight.

Follow directions on all medications, both prescription and over-the-counter. Make sure your pharmacist and any doctor prescribing for you know that you have a liver disease.

Talk to your doctor about any herbs or supplements you're taking since some can be harmful to your liver.

Exercise

The amount of exercise that is ideal for you will depend on factors such as previous fitness and health levels, degree of liver damage, other conditions you may have and any surgeries that you may have had, particularly recently. We encourage people to find the level of activity that optimizes their current health and fitness levels. Specialist physiotherapists may provide some useful individual guidelines. Some Medicare funding may be available to you via your GP.

A PSC patient may do anything from running a marathon, to in bed strengthening exercises. If you can, just keep moving.

Mental Health and Wellbeing

Being diagnosed with a chronic and often progressive illness can be devastating and take time to come to terms with. There are many natural and healthy responses to this. Always be kind to yourself as you learn about your new diagnosis. Don't expect to know everything straight away. Seek out support – family, friends and health professionals. Try to identify what help you need from them and accept that help when it is offered. Learn as much as you're able to about PSC and develop and understanding how the overall view fits in your scenario. Ask your doctor questions and find reputable sources of information online. There has been a lot of development in our understanding of PSC over the last 10 years, so be mindful of how old information is too. Importantly, find strategies to deal with the situations you face, and implement them as much as you are able.

Some research suggests that 28% of people with a chronic illness will also suffer from a mental health condition, with chronic pain increasing it's likelihood fourfold. It is not surprising then that many people with PSC have a co-existing mental health diagnosis. PSC may threaten your independence, ability to study or work, place financial strain on you and put strain on a relationship or even make a relationship difficult to start. Having a rare disease with sometimes invisible symptoms can lead you to feel misunderstood and disconnected from family, friends and even health professionals. Whether you have PSC in early stages and no other complications or you have multiple health issues and severe or end-stage liver disease, there are some things you can do to help you manage these conditions.

While these things are bound to cause a level of stress, anxiety is a condition that goes beyond that expected feeling of stress or worry and becomes more relentless and affects your quality of life and even ability to do things. People express their anxiety in a variety of ways – phobias or panic attacks, distressing dreams, fixating on issues and worrying obsessively about them.

If you think you are experiencing anxiety it is important you seek help as there are therapies and treatments that can improve anxiety significantly. Your GP is a good place to start, or websites such as Beyond Blue have helpful tips. You cannot make your condition go away, but you can manage your response to it.

Like anxiety, depression goes far beyond being sad. Depression affects how you feel about yourself, how you view the world and it's situations. It causes you to look at any problem you have through a magnifying glass. PSC is big enough on its own, we don't need a magnifying glass!

If you have lost interest or no longer find pleasure in the things you used to, or are unable to find new things that engage you, you may be depressed. Having PSC can have a real impact on your physical ability to do things, or it may be the thought of what might be to come, that has triggered depression in you. Whatever the cause, reach out to professional help and friends and family. Depression can be successfully managed in most cases. Building coping strategies and connecting with others who understand all form part of a potential framework for your management for mental health issues.

It is common to see symptoms of Post-Traumatic Stress Disorder (PTSD) in patients (and parents in the case of children) who are transplanted. Although not usually seen as a comprehensive disorder, these symptoms are important to treat for the obvious reasons of wellbeing as well as having some special considerations in transplant patients. One key feature of PTSD is the avoidance of things that remind you of the traumatic event, for example, taking your immunosuppressive mediations may remind you of the event so you don't take them. This of course brings it's own dire consequences.

A liver transplant for most people with PSC is a relatively anticipated event. While we may not know when we receive a transplant, we do know that it is imminent, giving a period of time to develop strategies to help in preventing PTSD. Research has also explored the concept that some level of stress in this setting actually provides space for growth and resilience.

Overall PTSD is a complex disorder, but if you feel you are experiencing any symptoms seek help early to enable you to manage it most effectively.

The key message about looking after your mental health is to seek help. At first from family or friends and support groups, but do not feel you cannot seek professional help. Finding a psychologist who specializes in the mental health of patients with chronic illness should give you a solid starting point for recovery.

Education

For those with PSC who are still trying to study, whether you are in primary school, high school, TAFE or university, if you need some additional assistance or allowances there are some avenues to follow.

Most institutions have education support who can help you navigate through the process, however, depending on your needs, you will need to actively engage these people and work closely with them to ensure your educational opportunities are maximized.

Like claiming disability pension, your diagnosis alone will not be enough to secure support. You will need to identify how your illness is affecting your ability to learn and what assistance or modifications you require to optimize your education.

Employment

With perhaps a few exceptions, a diagnosis of PSC itself shouldn't stop you from doing any job you want. However, depending on disease progression and what other illnesses you may have, you may find you need to temporarily or possibly permanently, modify your workload.

For some, even in the earlier stages, fatigue can demand the need for work modifications. More manual jobs that are physically demanding may put additional pressure on you, though there are many who can manage very demanding jobs. If you are affected by fatigue you may need to reconsider your hours or style of work.

Some jobs will require you to produce medical documentation to state that your disease in its current state and foreseeable future, is not expected to limit your ability to perform the job. Entering the police force may require something like this for example.

If you are employed or seeking new employment, it is the employer's obligation to make reasonable adjustments or to work with you to find a balance in a position you can manage. Both employer and employee have responsibility here, so consider the job you are being employed to do and if that can be reasonably adjusted to allow you to continue, or if it has become too much.

Work-Life balance becomes tighter with a medical condition. If well you will still need to attend medical appointments, and if you are more affected by symptoms, working long hours may take from your home life more than could previously be accommodated for. Finding your new, often ever-changing normal will bring you the best outcomes at work and at home.

Travel

People with PSC travel all the time. The key to traveling with any chronic illness is planning! While spontaneous trips may be a thing of the past, they don't have to be completely lost.

Things to consider when traveling include:

• Medications

• Ensure you have a good supply for the trip or easy access to top up while you're away.

• Consider taking a letter from your doctor outlining your current condition (your last specialist letter may be enough), in case you need to present to an emergency room somewhere.

• If you are flying you will need a letter to support your need to carry your medications as carry-on luggage. And ALWAYS take your medications with you on carry on. Any requirement for needles should also be stipulated in the letter.

• If you have any special needs for your flight, for example, wheelchair assistance or medical devices such as oxygen etc, let the airline know early.

• Consider where you're going and your state of health. What medical care might you need, and how will you get it.

• Discuss immunisations with your GP, and/or specialist travel doctor. Make informed decisions on the safety of locations in this regard, and which immunisations are safe and allowable for you to have. Do this well ahead of your trip especially if you are going to areas of high risk where multiple immunisations are recommended.

• Make lists! Plan, plan and plan a little more. Taking everything you need will help you enjoy your time away.

Fatigue Management

Fatigue in PSC can occur at any stage of the disease. Optimising any possible medical management can help, such as ensuring your vitamin and mineral levels are within good range, including your iron levels, and ensuring any treatable condition is treated, particularly any inflammatory or autoimmune condition.

Beyond that some more practical tips that might help you manage your fatigue include:

• **Listening to your body**: finding a balance between rest and busyness or exercise can be tricky. Knowing when to push a little and when to rest is a skill you can develop over time. Exercise and rest are both vital. Don't feel guilty about finding time for either.

• **Diet:** a healthy diet and maintaining good hydration may boost your energy and ability to concentrate.

• **Knowing your limits:** if you need to adapt your work hours see if your doctor can write a supportive letter to your employer. Take time off when you need to. And "budget" your energy so you don't miss out on the things that are most important to you.

• **Accepting help**: if your friends or family offer to help you out with things, it's ok to accept. Think about how you feel when you are able to help someone else, and allow someone to feel that way when they help you.

Liver Transplantation

1063 children and 4827 adults received a liver transplant between the first Australian transplant in 1985 and the end of 2017. As a rare disease, PSC makes up only small numbers of our national transplant cases. 8 children have received a liver transplant for PSC and 468 adults. Of the adults, around 30 have experienced recurrent PSC and required re-transplantation. The data collected to date shows our centres as world-class in their transplants with excellent survival rates.

The Australia and New Zealand liver transplant organisation collect data on each of our transplant centres. People are geographically allocated to their centres, of which most states have one adult centre, and some have an affiliated paediatric centre. In general, each centre accepts donor organs from its own region, however, in some extreme instances, a donor organ from another state may be allocated to someone. A region generally covers a whole state and may include a second state.

The decision and work up:

The decision for transplant is not one made lightly and is an important stage of the PSC journey for many people. Mixed emotions are common, fear, anxiety, joy, relief, among a few. If your doctor refers you to the transplant team in your region it is because they feel your liver is no longer functioning well enough and a transplant is a good option.

The transplant team is a multi-disciplinary team of hepatologists, surgeons, specialist nurses, radiologists, dieticians, psychologists, physiotherapists to name a few. Your "work up" will include meetings with some of these people as well we appointments with a number of other specialty doctors such as cardiologist and renal physician, who will order a further series of tests to fully evaluate your health and pre-empt and treat any foreseeable issues to transplant.

The preparation time:

I prefer not to use the term waiting….because waiting implies that you're sitting around doing nothing.

Once you're listed for transplant you have the opportunity and responsibility to be in the best possible shape you can be in, both physically and mentally.

Ensure you attend your appointments and manage your medications as prescribed. If your care is being shared with your regular hepatologist and the transplant unit check they each know what is happening in your case.

If you're not able to tolerate much exercise, find something you can tolerate. Finding an enjoyable physical activity, even if very light weight, will help you stay in better physical shape and improve your mental state. Even walking out to the letterbox can be an activity!

Keep living your life. You may have some physical restrictions that you have to work with but keep doing the things you love if you're able. Don't give anything up just because you're on the transplant list.   Go out for dinners and shows……even short holidays, so long as you stay within the parameters outlined by your transplant centre.

The surgery:

Be ready for a "dry run". You might get a call only to later discover that the liver is not viable, or not the best match for you. As heartbreaking as this is, try to focus on the fact that you were called, your time is nearing.

Once called in you will be prepped for surgery. The transplant team will have gone through this with you as part of your workup. Liver transplant surgery is a huge operation, but one that we have highly experienced and capable surgeons for.

The transplant is facilitated most often by the generous gift of organ donation from a deceased donor. Where someone has passed away under very specific circumstances and their family has bravely made the decision that their loved one's organs can be donated. Live donation, that is where a person donates a portion of their liver for someone, is sometimes considered, however it is not always suitable for a variety of reasons. It has most commonly been performed on children in Australia but is not a common occurrence in itself. If you wish to explore this option talk to your transplant team.

The recovery:

The recovery following a transplant begins in the intensive care ward. This can be quite confronting but is a highly specialised and monitored environment to give you the absolutely best first stage of recovery.

The time in ICU and then on a general ward will vary greatly. But each stage of recovery can be celebrated and enjoyed. While on the ward you will be educated about your immunosuppressant medications and any other medications you will need. You will remain closely monitored even once you return home, often having to return for blood tests and examinations in order to detect any issue early and deal with it.

Many people find they can return to their previous job and enjoy physical activities they have not been able to manage in years. Some even choose to participate in the National and International Transplant games.

Transplant is a highly successful treatment for most who undergo it, however, learning of the issues of immunosuppression must also occur. Lifelong medication to allow your body to keep your new liver is necessary. Your medical team will choose what is best for you and adjust to lower levels the further away from your transplant you get.

Unfortunately for a small number, PSC can recur in their new liver. This may or may not behave in the same way as your initial diagnosis, but your medical team will help you through this.

Alternative medicine

No alternative medicine treatments have been found to treat primary sclerosing cholangitis. But some complementary and alternative therapies may help you cope with the signs and symptoms of the disease. Talk to your doctor about your options.

Fatigue is common in people with primary sclerosing cholangitis. While doctors can treat some factors that may contribute to fatigue, your signs and symptoms may persist. You might find relief with complementary and alternative treatments that have shown some benefit for fatigue, such as:

Regular exercise done more than two hours before you go to bed, which can help promote better sleep

A well-balanced diet that includes fruit, vegetables, whole grains and protein

Stress management techniques, such as meditation and relaxation exercises.